TWELVE

YEARS

UNTIL

HEAVEN

My Mother's Memory Book

A journal written by Esther Haas

A family's journey with Brain Cancer

Written by Carmen Wurst (Haas)

I started this project two years ago. I had to go through all of Esther's notes. She wrote in such small fine printing. Her words would make me smile and cry. Sometimes I had to just walk away from this for days or weeks. Remembering it all was very daunting and draining.

In 1998, Esther was fifty eight years old when she was diagnosed with a Brain Tumor. She was seventy years old when she passed away in 2010. When I was forty four I was diagnosed with early Parkinson's Disease. This happened just three years after Esther was living with her ailment. The writing of this book was a huge challenge for me physically. Parkinson's is associated with tremors such as shaking. I typed this book with my left hand, finger by finger at some points. I am a right handed person. It was at times frustrating, debilitating and oh so worth it all.

But my focus is not on me this time around. Esther will get all the attention she deserves.

To My Family,

Richard, Rhea and Eric

Thank you for your patience, guidance and understanding while helping with the setup of this book as you knew it meant so much to me. For always being there for me when I couldn't be there for you. Your solid foundation gave me the time and opportunity to be by my mom's side when I wanted and had to be. For always having open arms for me to cry in after so many travels. To have you as my rocks is reassuring. You make me so proud. I love you.

ACKNOWLEDGMENTS: First and foremost: To my twin sister Karen.

Thank you for helping me remember the order in which all of these twelve years occurred. I have cried over the phone and had you listen to me tirelessly. There was too many times to mention. You have been the wind beneath my wings for fifty two years. Your devotion, commitment and dedication have been there for me always. You're not only my sister but my best friend. What shall I ever do if I lose you?

The University of Alberta Hospital and the Cross Cancer Institute in Edmonton can never be thanked enough. Their expertise in their fields, made Esther's life more extended. The work they all do for others is commendable.

The Peace River and Grimshaw Hospital deserve so much thanks for showing your tender and caring ways. You made Esther's last days a little brighter.

I know there were so many family, friends, Doctors, Nurses and people that tended to Esther over her twelve year battle with Cancer. We thank you from the bottom of our hearts.

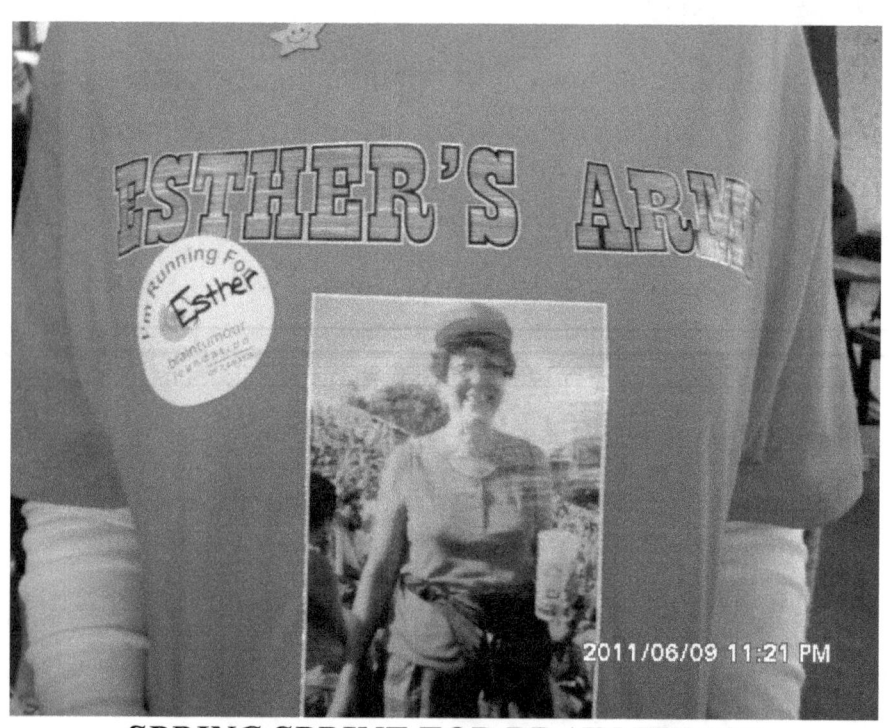

SPRING SPRINT FOR BRAIN TUMOR
FOUNDATION IN EDMONTON

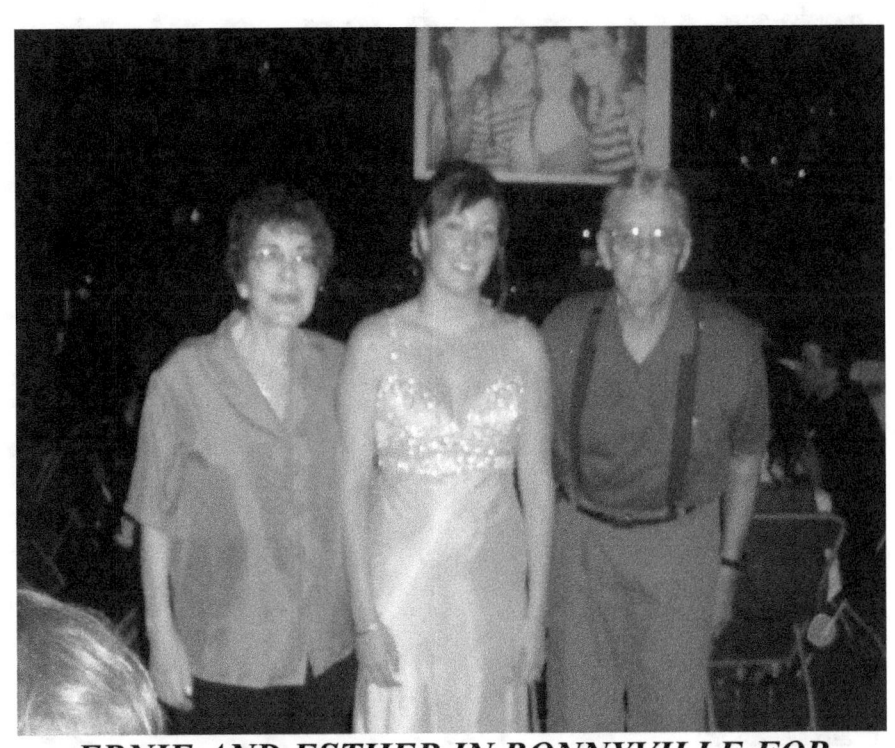

ERNIE AND ESTHER IN BONNYVILLE FOR RHEA'S GRADUATION

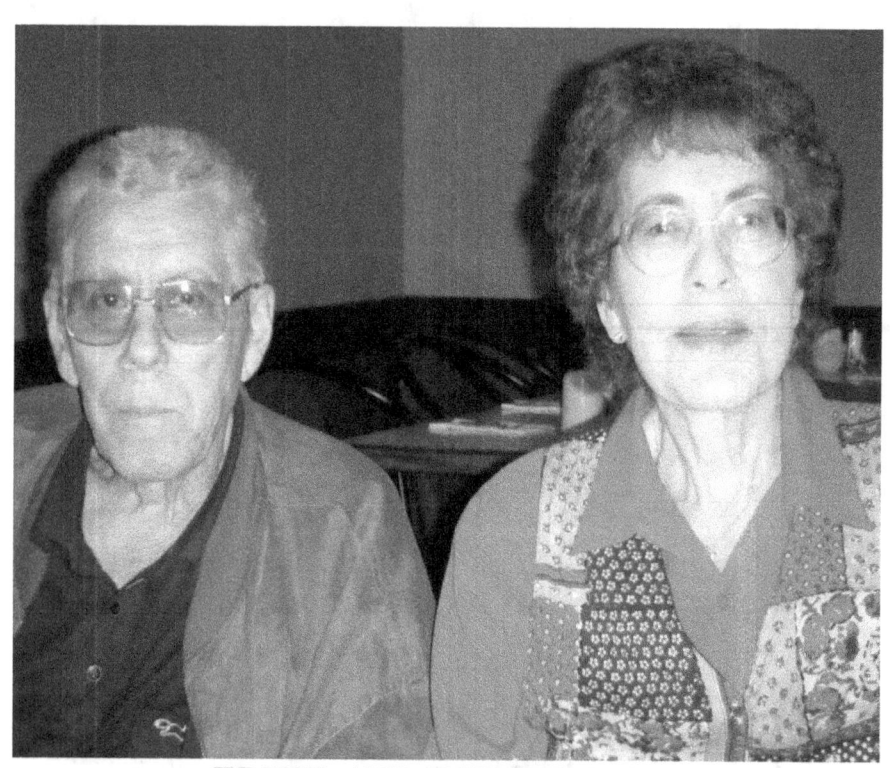

ERNIE AND ESTHER HAAS

THAT ONE WORD

How was I to know that one baffling long distance call was bound to change the course of my life forever? The desperation I felt at that particular moment in time was staggering. My mind let in all kinds of disturbances which left little room for any other thought process. The numbness became all too real and terrible worry floored my senses. The words that were being transferred to my mind were not coming through clear. How does one process the information I was given? With complete dread I was being told that my precious mother Esther apparently was dying.

With softness in my voice I expressed to Esther that I would very much like to put her words and mine on paper through a journal of time. She was impressed with my eagerness. I wanted her to write a memoir of her thoughts and feelings that pertained to her everyday life with Cancer. She did just that. For many of her twelve years battling Cancer she wrote religiously. When her right hand lost all mobility, she could no longer pursue this task, she had to stop.

I am going to open myself to you as best I can so you can experience the journey with my mother's Astrocytoma, Brain Tumor. My intension is to let you digest my opinions and statements. My truths are only going to surface from my firsthand sights and testaments. My medical terminology may not be correct or even knowledgeable in this field. I am not textbook savvy and don't claim to be. I apologize for any errors. I will just write from my heart and let you join the beat that I had to follow.

You will notice through this memory book that I speak of my mother and father as Esther and Ernie. I thought this might correct any confusion as to which parents I am talking about. I have inserted Esther's quotes in this memory book. Her recollections are vivid and poignant. Many thoughts of hers are very generic but others are extremely personal and completely raw in nature.

Our writing was a way both of us used to deal and heal with death. Her thoughts were just as much therapeutic for her as they were for me. Her printing was so small. The words were barely eligible, my eyes would strain just to make sense of her sentences. I would not give up. Her complete words were staring up at me, gnawing for me to finish what she had started. The extreme emotion was dreadful at times. I would catch my tears flowing down my red swollen face. I was prepared for moments like this. I would slowly shuffle away until I could face the truth again. The sadness would take over me plenty of times. There would be days when I could not continue until I was pacified again.

This Memory Book of Esther Stephenson (Haas) is a tribute to her and her family for being courageous in a time of need. Her lifetime must be told to help you understand who she was and how I have become me. Let the memories begin.

HAAS HOME

The property which Esther and Ernie, my parents, four split level house situated on was a particularly large lot for Grimshaw. The back yard was paradise for the children and grandchildren. The treasured back yard was landscaped with many poplar trees, willows and shrubs. The circular fire pit was at the beginning of the trees for shelter and convenience. It was a treat when the fire pit came alive with flames and smoke. The garden was planted with love and care and a mixture of vegetables from potatoes, peas, carrots to raspberries. Our children would go rushing to the harvest once it was ripe for picking. They would forage the various fruit and vegetables right off the vine or from the ground. They never found it necessary to clean their rewards as Grandpa Ernie would always say, "a little dirt never hurt anyone, and added to the flavor." Many serious baseball games were attempted in the spacious yard. Cartwheels and somersaults with bare feet on the new green summer grass would surely leave stains on the bottoms of our calloused feet. Mowing the huge lot was a certain challenge as there was a small incline near the back of the house. The extra-large cement deck was covered with white plastic sheeting above. This deck was grand for entertaining delicious BBQ's, Happy Birthdays, nervous Bridal Showers, loud Baby Showers, relieved Gift Openings, toasty Wiener Roasts and scrumptious Potluck Suppers. Juice was offered on hot long days of summer.

Coffee on the cool ones was common. This familiar deck became a place of comfort for all of us that had congregated there at one time or another.

ESTHER'S ROOTS

Esther's birth place was in Fairview, Alberta. She was born May Fourteenth, 1940. Her brother in law actually told her on her sweet sixteenth that she truly was birthed on May Thirteenth, a Friday. How he ever knew this information, she wasn't sure. Both of Esther's parents had serious health problems and bad luck was following them at this time. Supposedly Esther's mother Elizabeth put down Esther's birth date as the fourteenth while all other confusion was around.

Esther's eleven brothers and sisters were raised in the green hilly Montagneuse Valley, not far from Fairview. Their family homestead was spacious with a welcoming creek running through it. The land was cleared for a large log house. The wooden stairs in the home met with railing from up above. The sight looking down into the house was stunning. Farming was constant, fishing was necessary and hunting Moose all kept the huge family fed. They also had a Lumber Mill that was effective. Cattle, along with woolly sheep and wild geese kept the family extremely busy.

As a young girl still living in the family log home, Esther had a terrible fright one evening. She was walking up the dark wooden staircase with her oil lamp when she moved slowly in front of a slightly open window. The wind from outside pushed the breeze in and it caught the flame from Esther's uncovered lamp and brushed by her hair. Esther with panic realized the smoke and unpleasant odor was from her black hair being a blaze. She quickly responded to her dilemma and sat immediately on the step and smothered her sizzled hair. To stop any other future scares that night she closed the window steadfast.

Esther would attend the community school house for her education. Through the wind, rain and snow she would march. The distance to the small school was a huge endeavor. Many times she would encounter wolves and coyotes scoping and scouting her out. But even worse than those encounters, were the ones she had to deal with at school of the human kind. Her school had all the ages and different grades in the one classroom. When it was time for recess, the children would escape outdoors only to have fear brought to them by an older bully with a whip. He would send the whip through the air and it would connect with your skin and send pain shuddering through your body. Esther would experience this cruelty all too often. It seemed that there was no help in sight from anyone. Esther had enough of this madness and at recess when the whip came her way, she stood fast. As the end of the dangerous whip was just about to make contact she grabbed the hard material with her strong grip and then used the opposite end to do the same to her abuser. This fortunately would never happen again to Esther. This however mentally scarred her a bit I think. She mentioned this to me many times through the years.

She would recall it all with such vividness. She could still roll his name off her lips with judgment.

Esther's mother suffered with debilitating Polio and was wheel chair bound. Even though her mother was unable to walk she became pregnant with Esther and her younger sister. Her mother spent the majority of her life in the Peace River Nursing Home. Esther's older sister would live with Multiple Sclerosis and join her mother at the same nursing home. Esther's father was also unwell and had half his stomach removed in Edmonton. Esther's father passed away when she was just a wee girl of eight years. Esther was the second youngest child of the family. Her youngest sister died in March at two and half years old of Small Pox. Due to the health of her mother, and the absence of her father, Esther was placed in various sibling homes until adulthood. Esther being a devoted person guaranteed that her mother, sister and her brother-in-law would all be treated with kindness in their nursing homes. She continued to care for them all right into their later years. With her three family members living out their lives in long term care, Esther would purposely dedicate her time and effort to make positive that they were comfortable and secure in their surroundings. When death would call on each and every one, Esther was released from her duty which she had taken on so seriously.

ERNIE'S ROOTS

Ernie had a brother five years his senior. His brother was an Engineer and had a prestigious award given to him by the Governor General. He won the Order of Canada. His brother was a very fit and educated man. He had at an older age than most took his University courses. His brother and wife, along with their three children lived in Ontario. We rarely had the chance to see each other because of the distance between us. Ernie's little sister was fourteen years his junior. His tiny sister had orange hair like a carrot. She was beautiful in every way. She was physically stunning and had a personality which few did not gravitate to. At the young age of twenty-one she was taken all too soon by a motor vehicle accident. Ernie was so shaken by this tragedy. I can still recall the local police coming to the door and announcing the terrible news to my father. This was my first encounter with death. I was very young but still realized this loss of life was so conclusive.

Ernie always stated he was made in Germany and born in Canada. We kids always found that statement to be thrilling and exciting. His father and mother were German immigrants. His parents had strong German accents. His father was a short small framed man. His mother was a big boned, big breasted woman. They ate rye bread and sauerkraut, which I, as a child found disgusting. His father loved to watch wrestling. The Hart brothers were his favorite ones to watch. His mother had a real feather bed quilt that we children loved to play on. Ernie's mom had a sense of what would make us children giggle. She would sometimes, without warning take her false teeth out with a slip of her tongue and then slide them right back in. On our way to and from school, their house was along our path. We would stop regularly for sweets.

Grandma Haas was excellent at Knitting. She would produce beautiful sweaters for her children and others. Ernie was quit gifted with the knowledge of numbers. With this talent came the knack for strategizing and manipulating sequences. Ernie was able to assist his mother with producing patterns for her woolen crafts. The ensembles were very unique and worn with pride.

Ernie's father lived at home and tended his garden until he was eighty six years old. When he became ill with Leukemia he had a short stay at the nursing home in Peace River. The nurses would try to beef up Ernie's father by giving him beer to drink. The yeast would fill his stomach when nothing else was tolerable. What a nice way for the hospital to generate his fluid intake. I loved the gesture. My Grandpa took his last short breath with all family members in attendance. Ernie would not let any of us go notify the nurses that he had passed away. For ten minutes we waited. Ernie finally opened the hospital door and let the qualified nurses in to tend to his father. We as a family were there when my Grandpa passed on to the other side. It was so sad and yet so perfect for him to go so peacefully surrounded by his loved ones.

Ernie's mother was dealing with a disorder that many new nothing about at this period in time. Sometimes she thought along with her family that she was going a bit crazy. This foreign sickness was just starting to surface. The truth was this disease was incredibly vague in nature. Doctors and Scientists were just starting to get a tiny taste of the severity this could do to one's mind. Ernie would take her to specialists that would give clues as to what should be done with my Grandma. A lot of these doctors were seen at Mental Institutes or Asylums. People suffering from Dementia and or Alzheimer's disease were treated very differently back then. Despite protocol, Ernie brought her back home to Grimshaw. She was placed in an old folk's home in Peace River. There the family could visit with her often. She had quality care from professional nurses and doctors. She was made comfortable. Her memory was becoming so vacant. Ernie made the decision that we children should not attend to her bed side any longer. She did not recall who we were. It was very depressing, but Ernie had made the best decision and solution. She would perish years later with Ernie by her side. As like Esther, Ernie always had his parent's best interest at heart.

The Haas family, being of the German dissent put

them in line for some very mean and cruel practices. One Halloween my Grandpa had a Swastika spray painted on his Garage doors. Whether the crime was done by kids playing pranks, it didn't much matter as the damage was done. It had made Ernie's family feel outcast and unwelcome. A lot of people don't or didn't realize the significance of that image. My own daughter in the twentieth century in Grade nine or ten had a Swastika put on her passenger door with masking tape. She got in her vehicle and never saw it, as it was not visible to her. She drove through town none the wiser until a male friend of hers told her to look at her door. She was clearly upset and was shocked along with myself. Even in this day in age people are still using unnecessary tactics of racism.

THE ENCOUNTER

Esther was at an annual track meet when she was entering Grade Ten. She was practicing her high jump skills. Esther was rather talented at this sport as she would win first place in high jump in the Fairview Divisional from Grade Seven to Grade Nine. Ernie would with canter, dash in front of her every single time she went to distance the stretch. Esther also would play fastball with the boy's only ball team at school for the Divisional in Hines Creek. Esther became just a little fed up with Ernie's boldness. Ernie was the top male athlete in the Peace River Division.

They were to meet again at a high school dance in Berwyn. Esther was now in Grade Eleven. Ernie gallantly asked Esther for a date. A week passed by slowly for Ernie and then Esther accepted. A movie was their first interlude. Ernie fell asleep; Esther would wake him with a perplexed glare. They shuffled off to a dance nearby.

Their love blossomed and Ernie proposed to Esther while he was driving by the Fire Hall in Peace River on February Fourteenth, Valentine's Day. As you can tell, he was truly a catch. As their partnership gained momentum Ernie would show his romance through letters of love. My twin sister and I would find these words of devotion on paper late into my teens. We could not resist the temptation to every once in a while bring these letters of love to Ernie's attention. They were filled with such promise and commitment for the future. Their young love was to be forever and always.

THE MARRIAGE

Esther desired to get married in Hines Creek, Alberta. This wish was a difficult one as Esther no longer had a real home since Grade Nine. She was now eighteen and a half. Even though she was a legal adult she didn't have much to call her own. Esther was staying at her older brothers dwelling. The house was cool and the dust and dampness made her lose her voice almost completely. She had to take a month off of work at AGT (Alberta Government Telephones) as she was a Telephone Operator. June was the summer season Esther wanted her wedding. To have the rays of the hot sun and to feel the radiant warmth of summer was truly when she desired her union to become complete. With the farming season being on the top of everyone's list, Esther was to have their wedding on September Twenty Sixth, 1958. Her immediate family had a meeting and it was decided that Esther would have her reception in her brother's unfinished basement in the valley. Her flower arrangements were finished with artificial white and red roses. Esther arrived ten minutes late for the wedding ceremony as one of her nieces got her finger caught in the car door. Ernie along with the guests were puzzled with what Esther could be doing that would make her this distant. Ernie's mother was traumatized just a bit with the lateness of Esther's arrival. Their dearest friends and family stood by their sides when Esther and Ernie made a vow with God.

GRIMSHAW AND FAMILY

When it came to raising a family, Grimshaw was there destination. They chose to add to the Haas clan soon after they made their partnership in life. Their first two bundles of joy were little girls laced in pink. The next two babies that joined the group were also girls but happened to be identical twins. Ernie now had a family dominated of five females. The testosterone was surely lacking in this house. The twins were a welcoming surprise and punctually entered this world at ten: seventeen and ten: twenty a.m on March Eighteenth, 1963. Esther and Ernie were like everyone else, stunned with the blessing of the twin girls. In the days of no ultrasound there was no way for Esther to have known what was stirring in her large belly. Esther however did have a women's intuition, she always felt puzzled with this pregnancy. Completing the first delivery of one dark haired baby sent the doctor and nurse into mumbling in low speech away from Esther's hearing. She became nervous and frightened. Feeling exuberated and exhausted, these whispers from nearby were bringing out her worst fears, something in deed was wrong. The doctor came close to Esther. With urgency and encouragement he told her frankly that she had birthed one small baby girl and one more just like the first was going to announce its self promptly. Esther was thrilled with the best news, nothing was amiss. Each of the dark haired bundles weighed in at five pounds some ounces each. The girls were spaced three minutes apart. With this news Esther placed an urgent call to Ernie. The notice of this situation sent him to end the message with a giggle as this could not be so. Ernie was told directly that he most certainly was the proud papa of two more girls that happen to be twins. The two older girls would each have a baby to care for. Ernie now had five females occupying every corner of his house. These two girls with mirror like images would be each other's greatest support in life. They would grace the earth through adversity and prosperity together. Loneliness was never to be all that great. Their voices were always to be heard even through the miles apart.

GROWING UP

My childhood was blessed with the most positive memories. Creating and exploring were encouraged in our home. The outdoors was ours to search. With our senses running wild we could be gone for hours with friends. Adventures were ours for the taking. Our parents never really new exactly where we would travel. We would be with familiar friends that were known to them. If an emergency was to arise while we were chasing our spirits, there just was absolutely never any doubt that the group would stick together and find or get help. The trust in people was very prevalent and bred into ones actions. You helped your neighbor without expecting something in return. You used please and thank you, everyday, all day. Adults were persons that had lived and gained life's knowledge. Due to that fact, adults were shown they had authority. We considered ourselves lucky to have parents that gave us freedom to roam. We however never took that basic rule for granted. The lessons we learned were passed on from the elder to the younger. If you crossed the line and didn't respond to the advice you were given, the consequences could be severe. You got privileges for doing well and not by demanding or taking them.

As tweens the biggest deals in our sheltered lives were we ever going to see advances in our ever slowly increasing boobs. They could never seem to catch up to the popular girls. For some reason god was determined to make yours inch just a tad. The exercises of, "I must, I must increase my bust", just gave you sore arms and never any cleavage that you died to have. The bra that you so desperately wanted to get was the most uncomfortable over the shoulder boob holder. To get your period last, would surely be the death of you. To have to wear a large white piece of stuffing between your legs and then have to attach this to a bungee cord around your waist, definitely attracted me to this lifelong annoyance. But anything to put you higher on the social scale was a girl's wish. At fourteen, to drive with an older sibling was the start of change. The Driver's License at sixteen suddenly gave you freedom to dabble with independence.

As teens we knew little about real life but we tried to absorb what we thought was important. We understood that parents were trying to occupy our minds with goals and aspirations. We would have difficult situations come our way and were expected to sort them out the best way we could. These were lessons we would have to use in the future. However, until then we cared mostly about our fake and true girlfriends. Weekends were for staying and sleeping in late. Lazy evenings were spent with friends dreaming of the wonderment yet to arrive. A whirlwind of parties took up a lot of space on our agenda. The social news was lost if you dare miss one. Alcohol became so easy to access. Liquor cabinets were being raided on a continual basis. Hangovers were many. The male gender entered the equation suddenly. Time with friends became less and boyfriends were made priority. Falling in love for the first time at sixteen is not easily forgotten. Special times were made and still linger on in the mind from time to time. He holds a place in your heart. Eighteen makes you an adult. The bar becomes a rite of passage and initiation into adult hood. Your choices are now taken seriously. You have to think before you act. Your decisions could make or break your endeavors. The future is held in your young, unsure and doubtful hands.

Over the years, Ernie would see more drama, tears, laughter and love passed around between all of his women. The hormones were jumping and flowing continually. The peer pressure of friends was always up front and center and could cause major stress. Tears flowed from loves lost. Ends of life erased due to accidents. Death was immediate because of suicide. Age taking the old ones back to Heaven. God makes angels from those taken before their time. Births accepted by young mothers. There were marriages that had faltered under stress and others were continuing to build strong foundations. Jobs passed by because of lack of interest and ones taken because of no choice. Through all the sorrows came laughter? God created it so we could heal from pain and anger. Laughing until your face is a deep shade of red and your belly hurts can be magic. Laughter is a wonderful tool to make one forget and forgive.

THE START OF SOMETHING SERIOUS

One familiar day, Esther was taking her usual rapacious walk from her residence to the nearby local grocery store. Unfortunately to enter the business she had to cross a very busy highway that proceeded through town. Esther's home was on one side of an extremely spacious road and the store on the other. With patience she waited until it was clear to continue. Once she safely made it inside she made her purchases. While venturing on to the highway again she lost her footing and fell. Luckily she never hurt herself and the road happened to be calm with traffic. She picked herself up and continued home, feeling embarrassed and a little shaken. This was not to be her first encounter with the hard ground. She was puzzled as there seemed to be a force magnifying her awareness with her unstable stability.

Tonight was meal time at my eldest sister's home. We gathered there for kinship and to catch up on recent ramblings. My sister's blue prints for her house were set up just like Ernie and Esther's home. The four level split was popular in construction. The top level would contain the bedrooms and rest room. The next level would be on the ground. The kitchen and living room would occupy this space. The continual steps down would be your level just below the dirt but with windows still letting in light. This floor usually would consist of a family room, bathroom and laundry. The next drop down was completely darkened and used for storage or another rumpus room filled this space. My brother in law was preparing tasty mouthwatering chubby burgers and slender hotdogs. They fed us all too well. Our stomachs were filled to the brim.

On this particular evening at my sisters, Esther was placed on the end of the loveseat nearest me. She was sitting kitty corner to myself on an angle. When she would converse with me I judged that her left eye was focusing primarily on me but her right eye was gazing straight ahead. My words to describe this would be called a wandering eye. I observed this for a period of time. I wanted to be certain that her lazy eye was having difficulty searching me out. I vocalized to Esther my findings.

Esther relayed to me that her fierce headaches recently were hitting the inside of her skull with force. They were becoming huge sources of dread. Her prescription for glasses had been changing on a regular basis. To have proper vision was becoming a continual chore. Her recent behavior with disturbed eyesight and balance problems as of late gave her medical physician just cause to order a CAT Scan. This test was to be Esther's first primary look into her Brain. Esther was cleared of all issues that this scan could show. Translation of the CAT Scan determined all was correct.

With her guard up, Esther was searching for a reliable, functioning MRI (Mirror Imaging). She just went with her gut feeling that more searching had to be documented. Her local doctors were in agreement with her. Esther was in contact with a doctor from her MS (Multiple Sclerosis) days as president of the Peace River County Chapter. This doctor must have realized the importance of scanning and scheduled her in for an MRI as soon as possible in Edmonton.

On February Seventh, 1998, Esther and Ernie were in transit from their small farming town of Grimshaw, with a population of a couple thousand people, to the provinces capital of Edmonton which populated approximately hundreds of thousands. The duration of the trip would take five hours on mostly single lane highways. The town of Grimshaw was situated two hours from the nearest city of Grande Prairie.

Anticipation for the evening ahead was building as the day wore on. An annual community function was drawing closer with each passing hour. My husband and I longed to meet and greet friends, acquaintances and sponsors of the Ducks Unlimited event. The night was sure to be filled with smiles, laughter, drinks and the spending of ones money on unique draws. We enjoyed this particular event with our close friends. My parents, Ernie and Esther, would be coming to watch over their grandchildren as soon as her scheduled MRI was complete. Then we could thoroughly be captivated by the evening without the worries that come along with leaving your precious babies with sitters.

When Esther and Ernie arrived in the fast paced concrete jungle of Edmonton, they went straight forward to the University Hospital. They had plans for this evening and were on a tight schedule. They were to be back in Westlock for babysitting duty. This foreign place captivated you instantly. The hospital roof stretched up to the blue sky. The sure size of it was intimidating. These huge glass buildings were for ill people, not someone like Esther. People were everywhere, coming and going. You couldn't be sure who the professionals were. The patients wore scrub like clothing. The medical staff also wore various colors of dutiful scrubs. It was all very confusing for a lay man not from this land. There were so many floor levels, corners and hallways to get lost in. Couches and chairs for staff, guests and patients were placed everywhere. Nurses sleeping, having lunch and taking breaks were normal here. Cafeterias were dominated with persons in white, blue and green uniforms. Seeing people solemn and staring out into space was the norm here also. To be passing on words of sadness or glee was common. People were all waiting for news. Bad news, good news or news of any kind, was heard by all eventually. This was the place to come in search of answers.

I was becoming anxious for the arrival of my parents. I required a late evening out with my adult friends. My children I loved, but starved for some interaction with grownups. My parent's full day with appointments surely had to becoming to a close. Ernie and Esther would have to back track forty five minutes to our home in Westlock.

WESTLOCK

This was another small community thriving on cattle and farming. The town had a similar pace and routine as any other. The senior men would meet at the local restaurant to shoot the breeze with fellow old timers. The men would drink coffee until their bladders were full and ready to explode with the dark substance. The daily mail run was a usual. Children had to promptly get to the bus corner on time. Other kids had to get out the front door for their adventurous trip down back allies to meet up with friends and foes.

We had found that the move to Westlock was a wise choice. We were appreciative to adapt to the new surroundings with ease. It had been a stepping stone for the whole family. We were committed to making the adjustment as easily as possible. We had in the past traveled and moved numerous times. The packing and unloading of personal belongings was becoming a physical and mental chore for the both of us. Our young children where little and never noticed much about change as long as we were visible. Now they needed the security and familiarity of home. We were looking for a safe haven and believed we had found one. Our daughter was to start Kindergarten. Our son was entering Playschool in the fall of 1997. We were very fortunate that the kids met fellow students that summer and fall before the school year began. Friends and family would be able to make their frequent stops for pleasure and business as our home was in direct line with Edmonton.

The house we had purchased in Westlock was extremely unique. I am quite sure there is not another like it. The home was equipped with three levels. The top floor was fashioned with three bedrooms and one bathroom. There was wooden railing that was placed in front of all the rooms. You could see over into the grand living room. The drop from the top of the slanted ceiling to the bottom floor was not for height worriers. The main floor was down a flight of stairs, to the kitchen, living room and computer room. The main focal point in the house was its dominating fire place. It started in the living room and continued up the center of the house to the ceiling up by the bedrooms. It was just this beautiful formation placed by itself with no walls around it. The truly incredible rock face fireplace was beautiful to stare at. The natural stone that it was built with contained fossilized matter. Throughout the rock you could visually see and touch prints of all kinds. My daughter's room was decorated with bright purple walls. We were spontaneous and used scrunched up grocery bags placed in another color of purple and periodically dabbed that on top of the already done color. It turned out to be quite stunning. Her room was very spacious. My son's room was center and detailed with blue. Our room was off to the right of the stairs and was joined with the tiny bathroom. The yard was meticulous in nature. Ever thing had its place and was structured with such absolute precision. The special focal point was the gorgeous flower bed in the front yard. The bed was the length of the yard and had a dry river bed through it with white rock and flowers all around with a perfect bridge to cross. The mounds of scrubs, low lying flowers and majestic trees were groomed to preserve it all for another year.

CANCER ON OUR LIPS

As I sat in my favorite seat in my safe warm kitchen, the phones rings came to life. I answered it with calm and commonality as usual. Ernie's familiar tone came on the line. His voice however was a little scattered, nervous and had a under tone of worry. He just matter of fact stated that he and Esther would not be returning to the house that evening as planned. I, with annoyance quickly asked, "why". My vision of happiness was diminishing and becoming invisible with each passing moment. Ernie stated that Esther had her MRI as planned. It was seen by her Neurologist and M.S. specialist. The experienced doctor firmly stated in his words exactly "you do not have one trace of Multiple Sclerosis but you have a Brain Tumor." They had discovered and located this growing Tumor in the middle of her sheltered neck which was attached to her long flowing important Spine and her grand Brain. The official name for this Tumor was called an Astrocytoma, which means, (The star). Esther would be staying at the University Hospital indefinitely. She was to become an immediate patient. Ernie was in such silent turmoil that he was urged by the nursing staff to have a private moment away from Esther. Ernie was hopeful that his worrying would somewhat become controlled. Ernie would continue to document difficult and frightening news onto the girls back in Grimshaw. He would with slight and understandable confusion relay the direct line of procedures that Esther would program through while she was stationed at the hospital. Her first and very important measures were to withdraw and discontinue any prescription or nonprescription medication she was taking. Once all medicines were out of her delicate system, her blood would no longer be thin. This would of course become extremely significant with surgery. Your life saving dark red blood needs to be thick with nutrients and electro-lights, should a disaster occur. She would be put on meaningful steroids that would build up her resistance against potential threats. Esther then would proceed to have delicate surgery that would preserve her efficient and disturbed Brain matter. My impulse was to cry hysterically but I had to collect my nerves and not worry about me at this precise moment. My goal was to put on the big girl panties and assist Ernie with protecting Esther.

With Ernie's edging, I busily got Esther's needful belongings tucked back into her suitcase which had been dropped off the previous afternoon. Esther would without any such warning in advance have to be prepared to stay for several weeks at the hospital. Ernie drove back to Westlock with his mind overflowing with doubt and unsureness. Ernie on arrival to our house was full of anxiety and was in a rush to once more travel the rapacious highway. Leaving Esther to her own devises at this new environment that evening was troublesome. Our anguish was not leaving any space for release from today's findings. I became Ernie's observant passenger on this lonely stretch of pavement. The entire day of highlights was about to land on Ernie's shoulders with an unmistakable fury. This toll of knowledge was conveyed in his weariness. Ernie was so emotionally drained and spent. His shallow eyes and heavy lids went closed for a split second while traveling the busy highway. It was imperative now that the both of us get some much needed rest. The dark night would surely be full of night mares and terrors.

The resourceful staff at the hospital had arranged for Esther to have a single room in the Heart patient wing. That was to be the only single available room on such short notice. This would be her temporary home. The dim lights were on continually and made the small space eerie. This ward, for heart patients was only tolerable for Esther. Placed by her stainless steel bed was a monitor which connected to the nurse's station only steps away. There was special equipment that was so foreign to us all. Your senses were on alert here. The noise was only bearable. The nurse's station was never quiet. The lively men and women kept this area running smoothly. The urge to close ones eyes would be brief due to constant commotion. Esther never really found needed sleep for more than two or three hours at a time. A possible five hours during the day.

My three sisters with the disheartened news in hand were restless to get to Edmonton. Ernie also had the troubling task of notifying Esther's brothers and sisters with the harsh news. A lot of planning would normally happen for a northerner to venture out to the urban setting of the city. In a sudden case of do or die, you hope the important are notified and not forgotten. We were actually clueless as to the seriousness of the situation. Our ignorance was showing through. We along with the specialists were all finding out the gravity to her head trauma. She would require many more lengthy tests, uncomfortable x-rays and cruel blood and urine samples. Esther would be scheduled to see so many experts in all areas of medicine. The family was patient hearing all that was conveyed to them through frightened language from Ernie. Esther and Ernie needed the security of warm words of encouragement. The girls needed Ernie and Esther to understand that our arms were to be like giant wings and would protect them from any deliberate harm. This major interruption was urgent. We were bound by blood to bring on our powerful unity. Esther's ordeal was just beginning; the anticipation of probable unseen complications would make our bodies tremble but we would not show our doubts. The surface of Esther's condition was just being peeled away like layers of an onion. The center of my existence would soon revolve around this beautiful woman from this moment on. Cancer invaded my universe and made me a complete hostage. There were no negotiations or bargains made. Esther had a Brain Tumor and that was a fact. Cancer was surely going to be up front and center as long as she was living.

With the kids in tow this time we made a quite journey to Edmonton. We stepped into the University Hospitals main doors with sudden alarm on our faces. Your eyes gravitate to the strangers with sickness. You are entering a solemn building. There are numerous persons with colorful bruises, temporary casts, wheel chairs being directed by uncertain patients. IV's and catheters are inserted to ones skin with purpose. Managing the directions and not getting lost or confused is a challenge for the able bodied. The disabled have to wear their suits of amour to stay on track. This unique existence is functioning like a well-oiled machine. There is a place for all. Behind closed doors is where all the elaborate teaching, practiced chiseling and life changing strategies become the works of perfection. Everyone is here for a certain purpose. The reasons are unsure but you can feel the urgency in the air.

As the rest of the family arrived we joined troops to locate her room. We found Esther in the Unit for Brain Injuries. The posters and signage took me by surprise in this ward. Everywhere you glanced there was mention of Brain damage. The gravity of Esther's situation was becoming apparently clear. Only yesterday Esther was vibrant with laughter and smiling at my children. In a swift moment she had now become a new patient of this ward with a room number. The first seven long days in this unpleasant room were to be spent ridding her body of harmful toxins. Her daily medicine was to be flushed from her system. She was to congest the ever powerful steroids. They were preparing her slender body for survival. Her small frame would proceed to put on extra weight, build stamina and blood count for the operation ahead.

The present family occupied the handy hotel across the street from the University Hospital. We discussed the options of how we could proceed to stay with Esther through her trying and tiring week ahead. Through joint conversation we came up with a plan that would work for all. Some would justify missing work to stay in the city, while others would with unease continue home to Grimshaw and keep order. Every task we tackled big or small made the plan successful. We all had a role to play. No matter who accomplished what, it all made the big picture a little smaller.

A forty five minute drive to see Esther in the Brain Ward became common for me. You had to be prepared and pumped when you entered Esther's room. Her signature pink lips and polish were waiting as always. Esther would have her jacket on and full of vigor to move. Visiting days became one of lengthy walks around the perimeter of the hospital. She required the freshest of air in her lungs. She craved the heat of the sunshine on her face. With action all around, it made you feel like you were still apart of the living. The hours of being alone and lonely were depressing. We would lunch at Timmy's across the street often. Esther would swallow Big Mac's like she was a trucker. The Chinese food nearby would console her massive hunger, as she would digest every minuet morsel. The body was making adjustments quickly. Esther's hunger was increasing at an expected rate. With the steroids capturing her cravings, she could consume plenty. Her body was fulfilling the request made of her. The pounds went on but soon the hunger would disappear.

Esther waited for that week to end mercifully. The talk of a possibility of Esther's death was not a wanted discussion. There were many avenues that needed to be examined by both, Ernie and Esther. However reluctant they were, it had to be dealt with. Esther was to have major surgery. This procedure was delicate and very serious. The Brain being the controller of all circuits made just touching the wrong switch disastrous or even fatal. Her speech, mobility, understanding and memory could all vanish if the surgery was a failure. Esther would over the course of a week or so, have many hours of alone time to contemplate her morality. Constant chaos was floating in and out of her mind. Esther and Ernie would have to get all pertinent Wills and documents pertaining to her existence in order. They could not afford to be hesitant about her future.

SURGERY

Esther's surgery date was suddenly upon us. Her doctor placed the attending family in a confined room to discuss the schedule ahead.

This slow intricate operation was to take approximately five hours to complete. The Tumor was a large mass and dominated the Brain. The doctor indicated that the Tumors location on the Brain could be an issue. The medical doctor also had reservations about Esther's blood clotting consistently and how her body would react to Anesthetic. Esther was generally in fine shape for the pressures ahead but could be tested without notice. When the doctor would enter her skull, should the Tumor be too invasive, they would close the tissue on her head. Future options with the family at that time would be adhered to. The possibility of Esther's life being altered was becoming very real.

On February Twentieth , 1998 at eight fifteen a.m., Esther started her surgical procedure. We would become Esther's pray line for the many hours ahead. We would gather and be strong for her. Words at times would become scarce and elude us. With a glance to the right or left you were met with glares of worry. At times I would feel physically sick with dread. My eyes would search for the doctor, returning with news. Strong coffee would fill the void inside while you waited for words of comfort.

The Winter Olympics in 1998 became a blessing of

distraction on the television. Over the last week, Esther had enjoyed watching the perfection of Ice Skating in her quiet room as minutes ticked away. All of Esther's girls at one time or another had participated in the sport. We all watched nervously in the drab waiting room as little fifteen year old Tara Kapinsky won gold. How I wished Esther could have seen this display of excellence. She would have been thrilled. This little skater filled our hearts with confidence. At twelve forty five p.m. Esther's operation was complete. Maybe miracles could happen twice in one day. One gold won and one life saved.

Esther was in critical condition in the Intensive Care Unit following her operation. She would be stationed in this ward for seventy two hours. If her Brain was to swell it would happen during this damaging period. The attending doctor relayed the procedure to us. When her skull was cut open, they concluded that seventy five percent of this Tumor was imbedded in her Brain. This meant that the other twenty five percent was successfully removed. With Esther not being any of the wiser, her hairless skull was stapled shut where her incision had taken place. The nurses were trying to have a slight conversation with Esther. She was sedated but slowly coming too. Esther was asleep but thinking, "I hope I don't wake up in the middle of all of this." She registered her family through blurred vision as she was not capable of wearing her glasses. "Am I alive or dead," was the question she wanted to know, as everyone seemed so serious. Esther could plainly hear others and their painful calls. She slowly became aware of her surroundings. She wanted to certainly see every one of us. Tiny scared steps of direction were taken through this terrifying unit. Tubes were running in every direction, monitors let out interrupting tunes constantly and the very sure nurses seemed threatening. We would double up and take this panicked walk to Esther's bed side. She talked in a soft clear whisper. Her swollen head was bandaged. The top of her delicate fractured head was covered. With direct and precise words she relayed the message that she wanted us to promise her we would discontinue smoking. With gladness in my voice and gratitude in my heart, I of course complied "yes." The surgeon with distress wanted Esther to be placed elsewhere in the hospital as he did not want her to become depressed. This special section of the Intensive Care ward had four patients and two nurses. Esther had four tubes invading her body. Every two hours the skillful nurses would roll Esther from side to side so she would not stiffen. Esther was getting very minimal sleep. On her last night in this ward she would have to remind the nurses of her pain medication every four hours.

Esther was transferred to a unit where she would start her gradual healing. As her incision was pooling too much blood inside her head a tiny opening at the base was left for the fluid to escape. I was preparing and bracing myself for my first visit with Esther since her placement away from I.C.U. I was slowly but intentionally pacing to her bed. The back of her small frame and head were up against a window that was facing me. She was now not wearing any restricting bandages. The wet tears started dribbling down my pale face. The shock of her bald neck and head, the length of her nasty incision and the abundant staples captivated my stare. I took a gallant breath. I entered the room quickly and placed a tender kiss on her cheek. I dismissed myself so I could prepare Ernie for the intense sight.

POST SURGERY

Esther was to receive many beautiful flower arrangements through her stay at the hospital. Many of these tokens would have to be dispersed elsewhere unfortunately. The fragrant blossoms were too powerful for the patients in the Brain Unit. Esther sent me and my twin sister home to Westlock with a gorgeous bouquet of hers one evening. As we were gingerly moving down a quiet hallway, a man busily rushing by us made a sudden stop right in front of us. He, in a panic asked the two of us questionably if he could buy our visible flowers. He stated that his friend had just been transported to this hospital. She had injuries to the head from a horse accident. He mentioned that the store was closed on the lower level. He relayed that he might not get the chance to deliver any before he would have to depart. My sister and I concluded that Esther would have graciously given him her flowers. This total stranger required my address so he could return the planter that had accompanied the bouquet. When the gift had completed its cause I would indeed receive the planter back true to his word.

Esther would be dismissed from the University Hospital and would be residing at our home in Westlock over the following ten days. Ernie would accompany her for a period of time. The girls returned home with heavy hearts. Ernie would ask my kids right from the start of Esther's stay, "Ok, we should all get a look at Grandma's wound." My son being seven and very assertive was captivated by the strategy of it all. My daughter however was frightened by the sight and didn't care to comply. It became apparent that some strangers, friends and family would all react differently to this predicament. One day in particular, my son was constructing a building with his ever favorite Lego. Esther was reading intently on the couch. Esther's grandson gently and clearly stated to her, "It's ok to cry if you want." Even the smallest of beings could be affectionate and compassionate.

With each day passing Esther's incision would gradually mend. The mobility of her neck could stretch more easily. Her lengthy scar would start from the middle of her left ear to the bottom of her neck. She was very conscious of her visible staples. She was becoming restless, with the long days being indoors. Today I made the decision that we would venture outside. Being February in Alberta, the crisp air was very fresh. She was unprepared along with me as to how the public would react to her misfortune. We gathered ourselves up and drove to the nearest ladies store. With many stares and some smiles of kindness we purchased a burgundy hat. When placed just so this soft felt hat concealed her staples. A day of being in charge of her situation was therapeutic for Esther. She could still feel feminine and not on display.

Today Esther was to have her staples removed. We had an appointment with the local Doctor's office in

Westlock. The nurse that was to do the procedure of removal was nervous once she saw what was revealed. The nurse steadied herself for the task at hand. The sturdy and strong staple remover did its required job. As I watched, I would cringe with every squeezed pull. The dried blood and skin had started to adhere to her flesh. The tightness of the skin forming around the staples was diminished. The tracks that gathered were still sensitive. The air would now cleanse the area. Esther was worried that the qualified nurse would lose track of a single staple. The procedure was complete. The nurse and I both felt extreme relief and paused with a huge sigh. Esther was direct and orderly with this nurse. "Count the staples in front of me one by one please." The nurse complied. Twenty nine was the correct count. Esther was pleased and at ease. She never wanted to experience that gut wrenching feeling again.

Esther took a moment to digest every minute up to this point. She was an ordinary woman living in a sudden nightmare. She had entered a hospital a vibrant independent saucy woman. She had made an exit out a fragile and confused person. She was now totally dependent on her small army. We would transport her to appointments, deliver medicines, transcribe schedules and monitor her bowel movements and measure her intake and outtake of fluids. She felt blessed to have us all rally around her. She would get frustrated and angry with the loss of herself. We would have to be patient and understanding. The verbal beast in all of us would be tested time and time again.

RADIATION TREATMENTS

With the metal staples favorably discarded. The radiation treatments were the next to take battle with the unforgiving Cancer. My husband would commute with Esther to Edmonton for her first shield fitting. Once placed in a secure room, Esther would be put in an embarrassing situation. Esther was told to, "take your shirt and bra off." Esther stared at her son-in-law with surrender in her eyes. She knew my husband would be discreet as possible. He would show compassion and empathy for this woman that was just trying to stay alive. The plexi - glass shield would be measured for a mask. She would eventually lie on her stomach with the mask situated over her face. She was not to move. The laser would direct the radiation to the Tumor and purposely not to her spine. The mask was to protect certain areas. The shield would keep the radiation from going through to sensitive places that could be damaged.

I took the ever timely task of getting Esther to her next MRI. I sat patiently in the small crowded waiting area. Esther was in the changing room slowly putting on the universal scrubs. I scanned all the faces sitting in the nearby chairs. The worried looks were familiar. Esther came and sat closely beside me. She was so exhausted from all the current medicine and nights of restless sleep. She quickly and peacefully fell into a deep solid slumber. Her head slightly fell onto my ever ready shoulder. This moment took her into such a relieved state that she suddenly and loudly presented snoring. Various people were glancing in my direction. I would not and could not force myself to bring her out of solitude. I felt so protective of her at that moment. My tears were being forced not to surface. I would be the rock she needed right now and let her relish in the comfort of rest. The somewhat irritated patrons would just have to deal with it. As long as I was present, Esther could saw those logs as loud as she wanted.

She was to require one more fitting for her shield as scheduled. Esther had been placed on Steroids before and after surgery. That increasing appetite she developed was from the medicine. Her face had become increasingly round during those weeks. The mask was unbearably tight. She was not able to tolerate the snugness for any length of time. A new mask was to be made to accept her difference in shape and space.

Esther's vision had faltered drastically. The enlarged Tumor had been pressing on her optic nerve in the right eye. This was causing double vision. To correct this problem, she was given a Prism to wear. It was placed on the center on her right lens of her glasses. This basically was a decal. She was forced to concentrate her focus to the center of her glasses. She would have to use this device until radiation treatments were finished. The eye would be treated in the future once sight was determined by the specialists.

From this point on Esther had been transported to the University Hospital and the Cross Cancer Institute by family members. Now the squad was to dismiss and head dutifully home to Grimshaw for a period of time. Esther was now being placed under my watch. I was however not an avid city cruiser. My knowledge of these joining streets and avenues were not stationed in my mind. I had always been the silent passenger that never paid much attention to detail. I had certainly not made any real distance on my own. Ernie had shown me firsthand how to navigate to the University Hospital. Following his instructions and directions, I cautiously advanced into the city biting my already short nails and grinding my teeth continually. I proceeded down the three lane street hyper ventilating. The center lines seemed the logical place to proceed. I passed through nerve wracking traffic circles, overcrowded bridges and past many landmarks. I finally turned left into the underground parking as instructed by Ernie. This is where I was advised to stay during my visits. With sheer terror in my over focused eyes, the parking sign read FULL. I was about to panic but I had survived the journey thus far. Where was I supposed to park now? I would not fail so quickly. I scanned my surroundings. The moving people seemed to be a massive swarm. Tall buildings were blocking out the sun. Street lights changing color and signs posted with too much information. My sight veered across the street to a huge lot. With hope in my sight and my hands shaking, I maneuvered with slight confidence to the parking yard across the street. Once I was placed, my rapid pulse began to slow. This would be my first of many identical courses repeated to the hospital. With each solo mission my determination and confidence grew in bounds. When under pressure it is amazing what one can accomplish.

The residence at the University Hospital became Esther's temporary home for six consecutive weeks. She was a bit intimidated by facing the unknown alone. She was to take the next steps in facing this intrusive Cancer. The schedules and demands were daunting but she would have to comply. She was anxious and unsure of exactly what to expect at the Cross Cancer Clinic. Her emotions were in overdrive. Her scarred Brain had to absorb many details. The total lack of sleep was draining on her fractured body. She would possibly get two to three hours of sleep at a stretch. Five hours in a day was not nearly enough time to function properly.

On March Thirteenth, 1998, at one twenty p.m., Esther inched her way on to the daily transfer bus. The Cross Cancer Institute being the destination for Esther's first round of Radiation. The route would take approximately ten minutes to complete. All the patients exited the tiny bus and gathered to the entrance for the ritual to commence. Esther would navigate with the crowd to the waiting area. She concluded with observation that many persons in the clinic had a disturbed gait of some sort. She calculated that she herself made a portion of that group. The radiation would be a welcome intruder to battle the Cancer but a hindrance for the rest of the sensitive body. Esther's hair would thin with the increased Radiation over her neck area. The abundant weight her body had gained intentionally would now start to disappear. Her large appetite was depleted. Her body would go into survival mode and use those extra pounds when needed to supply Esther with nourishment. Her extreme fatigue would take her down like a bear in hibernation.

A routine would take place every Monday of Esther's six weeks of Radiation. I would dismiss myself from work and arrive in Edmonton at the hospital at 10:00 a.m. sharp. We would venture out for a casual lunch in the vicinity. With our hunger dealt with we would return and take the bus or walk to the Cancer Clinic. This became customary. This particular February in 1998 was an extremely mild winter. If the day was warm we would shuffle through the massive parking lot and enter the Clinic with rosy red cheeks. Esther relished in the fresh cool air. Esther would tackle her predicament and behave with simple grace. With the restricting shield in place, the laser pulse was penetrating the Tumor.

I nervously waited for Esther to complete her Monday Radiation schedule. I felt so ordinary as everyone around me seemed to be dealing with the extraordinary. While assessing my surrounding area I noticed a somber looking lady about my age of thirty five. I could just tell she was a patient by her facial expressions. Her scared mother was holding her hand and sniffling quietly. I am certain the young lady felt some resentment towards me. Here I sat among them with my invisible security blanket enveloping me and my future. She was probably so unsure of her destination in life. Would she survive this huge hurtle or would she slowly drift away like so many before and after her. The impact of this woman hit me like a train wreck. My mother and this young stranger were committed to brave this war on Cancer. They had no choice but to continue and cope with their outcomes.

Esther brought her ever loved sewing machine to the residence at the hospital. Over the years she would create eight individual pieces of art. Each grandchild would receive their individual quilt. She would cut and compile material to decorate with. Each quilt was designed specifically with each child in mind. Some were naturally girlish, pink and feminine. Others were more bold and whimsical. The special gift would in any case resemble your life in material. Each pattern cut with a reason in mind. Each fabric was used with a sense of purpose. If your family pet was a small, curly haired animal, it was displayed with importance. This task at hand would keep Esther's mind occupied during times of quiet. She could become focused with the delicate nature of the organized project. The negative memories would escape and disappear. She would skillfully attend to her only grandsons quilt during this trying time.

Esther's thirtieth Radiation treatment on April Twenty Ninth, 1998 came to a halt. Five days a week of continual pressure was pleasurably final. The six weeks of repetition was gladly finished. She was now free from the confinement of the hospital and Cancer Clinic. She could pack up her belongings from the small room which had heard so many prayers and tears. Esther would say, "God bless and God speed," to her fellow cancer comrades. She could taste the freedom just outside the double doors. Her imprisoned body was urgently ready for the future. This residence which had housed her would not be missed. She was to be embraced in the arms of her family very soon. Modern medicine had dished out all they could for her at this point. She had given her all to those who had demanded it. She had the right now to be selfish. She had shown massive courage in the face of darkness. She was to ask her mind, body and soul to cooperate at this time. She required this break from all things and needed to get back to some normalcy.

HOME SWEET HOME

Ernie was to take on many responsibilities when Esther arrived at their home. He was now to become the care giver. This role reversal would have to be tolerated. The house that was baby proofed decades earlier was now being adapted for an ailing adult. The demands made upon him would be challenging. He was to reinvest his energy in her wellbeing. They would have to explore this new plan of survival many different ways. The dramatic changes in their lives would be constant. The united front would be forced and tackled on many levels.

Ernie and Esther's three daughters would become an extremely important resource for the team. Ernie would undoubtedly be called away for work at a moment's notice. He could be gone as long as a couple of hours or as lengthy as a full day. The pressure was then put on the girls to coordinate and negotiate in times of caring for Esther. The girls had assured Ernie he was not alone in this venture. The consequences of the surgery would put all of them on standby. The girls would leave their families to make positive that Esther was in capable hands.

The home was made secure for Esther when she had alone times. The staircase leading down to the lower level was to be blocked off so there would be no chance of falling. A safety rail was attached to the bed for reassurance. The bathtub lift became urgent and most useful. Esther would need that immediately because of her balance situation. A taller toilet seat was recommended. A fork and spoon with weights in them made eating less of a chore. A walker would make her travels in and outside simply easier. A wheelchair that was a nuisance to fold, absolutely made her life and the care givers more bearable. The local home care facility graciously gave these items to Esther on a need basis.

Esther's arrival home greeted her with anticipated nausea. She had suspected it would come but not with vengeance so strong. The daily reminder of her prognosis was ever present with this continual feeling of dread. Sleeping pills were administered as her mind would not absorb the facts. Each day the undeniable quenching of thirst due to medication was on her tongue. The sickness from Radiation was taking a toll on her appetite. Certain medicines would consume her with tiredness. She would take heated bean bags to bed with her because of the sharp pain she was facing. She became cold like an icicle. In the middle of hot summer days she was wearing long johns under her pants. The freezing shaking would tire out her muscles. She would get the sensation that a million little needles were prickling her. She could digest seven pain pills in a day alongside with her other required medication. Also the negative thoughts were on her mind. To be optimistic about the future was tough. The tension and fatigue were very hard on her physical and mental state. With time some of these setbacks would diminish and fade but others were right there to take over. These alarming side effects would last an entire year.

Esther was glad to be in the familiar surroundings of her treasured home. The luxuries of her comfortable queen mattress, with soft warm blankets were a gift. The right fluffiness to her pillow was accepted with pleasure. To the sudden left of the pale yellow bedroom was a one of a kind laundry shoot. As children we had practiced placing our slender bodies in the precise location to drop without hurting one's self. If done correct, the ride down two flights of stairs became a thrilling drop. We would of course never tell of our adventure. This was a secret only the young were privileged too. I am sure Ernie and Esther were accustomed to our trials and errors though. Her pastel purple bathroom with two sinks was just to the left. She knew where the amenities were all situated and belonged. Down the long stretched hallway were entrances to two spare bedrooms. After a flight down, you embarked on the large living room which was privy to a major large window.

In the presence of her home she could finally take a short moment to ponder what was to happen to her now. The doctors with all their wisdom had given Esther and Ernie the prognosis of her surviving, two to five years. That damaging information was privileged to her immediate family only. Esther did not want the rumor mill to spread as that would surely happen on its own. She had always been a survivor of sorts. Her challenged up bringing had made her a force to be reckoned with. This time it would take all her positive energy to rise to this drastic occasion. She would become her own diligent master in the forces of reality. She would change what she could and try to accept what she could not. She no doubt would have days of anger and sadness of what she would miss along this unknown path. Esther would however tackle each day one day at a time.

The family's knowledge of this outcome of Esther's was unbearable. This small window and reference of time made me want to hold her soft small frame and never let her go. I could not contemplate my life without her in it. My mind would never drift to far from Esther. She was in my wrapped up thoughts constantly. Would she leave me now, tomorrow or a year from now? The not truly knowing of when Esther's demise would come was extremely damaging on the soul. To live your life was to maybe miss out on hers. The continual dread of each day passing was to make havoc of the new one ahead. My life had become a series of I shouldn't, I couldn't. What if we are not handy for whatever was to arise? It became normal to have this preparedness stamped in the back of our conscious minds. I always had a suitcase packed. I was ready for my sisters beckoning call. We were on duty twenty four hours a day and seven days a week. My family that I adored was in Westlock but my heart was beating with Esther in Grimshaw. I would learn to participate at a distance. My words of encouragement could not help when a physical body was needed. I would have to let go and put her in the capable hands of my sisters.

ERNIE'S SIDE KICKS

My twin sister and I would rise up early on Autumn Sunday mornings. With eager in our growing bones we would become Ernie's sidekicks for the day. These were the times when he would teach us to drive when we were thirteen or so. Our favorite spots were up in the Sulphur Lake area by Dixionville. Ernie would nervously guide us. He would spit out fast directions at one of us girls as we drove the GMC truck. While he scouted for Partridge we drove to the best of our ability. Ernie had his rifle or shotgun placed precisely out the passenger's window. With Ernie's eyes glued to the bush ahead he would whisper "stop" quietly. We would force the half ton to a sudden jolting brake. As we were extremely new to this practice, Ernie would often not be successful in his shooting targets. Our driving talents increased with practice which meant Ernie's shot would become more accurate. We were taught at a very early age never to kill a wild animal unless you were planning on using all of its body parts. The animal that was sacrificed should never go to waste. This message was instilled in us. Ernie's guns were not hidden from anyone; they were very visible to all. They were arranged on a gun rack in the family room unlocked. We were very sure of what damage a gun could cause and it never crossed our minds to challenge that thought. To touch this weaponry would call for serious consequences.

My sister and I spent many memorable hours with

Ernie and Esther in the tranquil lush green forests of Sulphur Lake. A lot of our Sunday's growing up was spent in the bush having wiener roasts and such. I always arrived with such anticipation and appreciation for these scenic views. We would just have a simple day of exploring the back roads and cut lines. We were taught to organize shelters from willows and full tree bushes. Soft leaves and greenery like moss could be used for flooring. The Blueberry, Saskatoon, Choke Cherry, Wild Strawberry, Rose Hip and Blue Bells could all be eaten in case of an emergency. You just had to know which berries were not poisonous. Ernie and Esther found it was important to pass this knowledge on as it was also taught to them as youngsters. I believe it was a necessity of their generation, like learning to swim or riding a bike. I have in return also passed those teachings onto my own kids. I hope that my children will continue the tradition of sharing nature. At times in one's life, the clearness of all things natural can make sense when nothing else does. To be back in the quiet of nature, makes us clear our heads and learn how to mellow from life's pressures. My own being would not be as fulfilling without the essence of Mother Nature. Just to roam the vast bush and taste solitude could be fulfilling. Every trip had a new experience in store. We investigated old trapper's cabins, wandered down creek beds and become dusty and dirty while searching it all. We enjoyed every stain made by the minute. Being mud from head to toe just always felt right. The earth made you feel welcome and alive at home on the land. Ernie and Esther may have had four daughters but were taught to be independent, strong sufficient women. The seven immediate granddaughters have the same strong will as their mothers.

Another Sunday spent at Sulphur Lake. This trip involved just me, Esther and Ernie. Ernie reluctantly stated, "I really hope we don't spot a black bitch today". Sure enough, what caught Ernie's attention in the short brush was a huge black/brown Moose. With the skill of a trained hunter, Ernie shot the gallant animal dead. The next inevitable task at hand was to start to skin the massive Moose before the generous meat went bad. Esther would with trepidation hold the long legs open at the rear. I with purpose held the other two lengthy legs at the front. Ernie would start skinning the tough hide down the center of the chest and stomach. As soon as Ernie sliced through the meat, Esther gagged with disgust. She sprang off to her right side and let go of the long legs which she was holding. With her sudden momentum, the gigantic Moose flipped closed instantly and jerked me with it. I was not prepared for this sudden action. With effort Ernie finished with the skinned Moose. Strong men from up the cut line had heard a shot and came to investigate. They pulled up alongside and assisted Ernie. They all helped with the lifting process of the heavy Moose. Ernie's truck now contained generous meat to be packaged. Over the years, I saw much wild meat shot, skinned, packaged and eaten. I became skilled in knowing when someone was feeding me wild meat.

A MAN OF MANY QUALITIES

Ernie had a very kind and caring heart when it came to animals of every breed. This is another trait we all inherited. We were rapidly bringing home lost or abandoned creatures. Rabbits, Kittens, and Puppies, all were brought home for inspection. Spring birds would clash with the clear patio door. Fall birds with fermented berry brains would try to dissolve through the hardened glass. Rye or Vodka was then present to put their tiny delicate beaks into the strong potion. This potent taste was sure to wake them from their daze. Needless to say each and every one of Ernie and Esther's children would have the unconditional love of a dog or cat present in their homes. Our pets have loved us and taught us more about loyalty than humans ever could. These true and honest animals have touched our hearts and placed smiles on our faces and giggles in our chests. These pets have become our companions and confidants. Ernie's teachings were heard loud and clear when it came to treating all with much kindness.

My first dog in my own home was a Terrier Cross with a Sheltie. Her name was Ginger and I cherished her with all my being. Where I went she was sure to follow. She became my shadow. Her presence was always welcome and made my days joyous. Her happy demeanor could only make you feel acceptance when you made an entrance. After twelve wonderful years with her friendship, she became ill and in pain. We put her down as I could not bear to see her in agony. It was truly one of the most peaceful and saddest days of my life. I was there when she slipped out of this world with a quiet sigh. I had her cremated. I miss her.

Ernie owned a GMC, Chevy, Olds car dealership in Grimshaw. This challenge to become sole owner and operator was a very big leap to take. Having a family of five counting on you to be the major bread winner of the family was a huge weight to hold.

All of Ernie's children at one time or another would be employed by working in the wash bay for the summer months. No special treatment was handed out. Ernie expected us to arrive on time just like everyone else. We would put in a hard day at work and feel good about it. Ernie was sure to teach his practices about the working world. A person rarely receives anything for free. You work hard and receive what is earned to you.

Ernie would own this business through much of my school years. With the economy starting to fail in those days, small businesses had a hard time trying to survive. You had to put more money on the line to sell more and work harder than ever before. With a sad heart Ernie had to close the doors to Haas Automotive.

I remember with that day came a puzzling statement to us from Ernie. "I am so sorry I let you guys down." That could have been no further from the truth. Ernie had always given us so much in material prizes but even more through his love and devotion as a truly great man and father. He was so worried we would see him as a failure. I saw him as a warrior and provider, and did what he had to do to survive. He is my hero, always.

When Ernie had the General Motors Car Dealership, he also sold Ski-Doo's. My twin sister and I were on these units every chance we got. Ernie would have two sleds at home usually for us to enjoy. Ernie would with purpose get us stuck and then make us figure out the details and plans of getting this ski-doo up and running. We would rock back and forth, use our hands as shovels and find any means possible to get this damn thing moving. These challenges were physically exhausting. Ernie wanted his girls to be confident that when we were traveling on our own that we could take care of ourselves. Ernie had taught us well, as we could without a doubt maneuver these machines as well as any boy our age. After school was a sure thing for friends to gather and go sledding. We would blast through the fields of powdered snow. Our eyes were always trained and strained to watch for barbed wire fences that would be hiding under the packed snow. The drainage ditch was the destination of choice. Slippery slopes covered each side of the huge dip. It became an accomplishment to stride over the crest in one giant leap. We would conquer the quest with many unsuccessful attempts. When all were tired of the jumping we would congregate in the close secluded brush. This group of close friends would use this place as a sanctuary away from uninvited guests. Our afternoons were spent with smiles on our faces as we had the real winter wonderland for the taking. We were busy being kids and loving every minute of it. We would have to head back to reality when the sky started to turn dark. We all kept a keen eye on one another. These times were enjoyed by all, as growing up was right around the bend.

FATHER, HUSBAND AND FRIEND

Esther was starting to worry about Ernie's health. He was a master salesman by day and a skillful farmer by night. He sold vehicles from his Chevy lot to strangers and return customers. All his energy was spent keeping both careers going. The hard living was starting to be noticeable. Ernie could be in better physical shape and he had his share of health problems. Ernie would always tease us by saying, "I am just a physical wreck." Ernie's back issues went back as far as I can remember. Over the course of years we children would give him various natural or bought remedies to try on his ever aching back. We would pressure him to try vitamins, lotions and attach electrodes to pulse his nerves and whatever else we could find in stores, T.V. and internet. Everything was just a temporary fix and not a permanent solution. Ernie was a hard labored working man and had the battle wounds and scars to prove it. Ernie is what people would call a man's man. He is one to never slow down even when his aching body would beg him to relax. This earnest commitment to finish tasks started has put him in jeopardy many times.

Ernie's role as father, husband and friend he would take very seriously. We always knew Ernie would be in our corner fighting for justice if need be. One regular school day along with my friends we decided it was a great idea to skip our scheduled classes. We all were sequestered at my friend's home for the whole entire day.

We relished in our freedom. No rules or assignments for the duration of this stay. I was having such a blissful time that I had not ventured home for lunch. Ernie with trouble on his mind thought I might be having issues with a particular teacher that I did not seem to reason well with. Being the helpful and supportive father that he was he marched over to the school looking for absent me. In his quest he encountered a realization that I had not attended any subjects thus far. When the simply perfect period came to an end I ventured home for supper. I was mystified that Ernie and Esther new about my where about. I guess my new haircut didn't give any clues as to my actions taken. Here Ernie had come to defend me against a tyrant in my eyes. I spent a good while glued to my room after that episode. Until I was much older I would ponder and wonder how they knew my actions. They always seemed to have eyes in every corner watching my moves. I understand that it was a form of protection on their part. Small towns they say, know everything about everybody. To a degree it is so true.

Ernie and Esther truly cared about the less fortunate. Over many decades I would see them show acts of real kindness. Esther was President of the Multiple Sclerosis chapter for many years. They would arrange huge Garage Sales and assist with Trail Rides to raise money for the crippling disease. Ernie would be most helpful to a common and familiar man in town with food, clothing and shelter through spells of hardship. An old family friend lived in a cabin in the middle of the dense forest. He was always Ernie's concern. Ernie would make sure he survived draughts, floods and winter storms. I would be Ernie's participate on many junctions that only he would make an entrance to.

In my early years Ernie occupied a tow truck. He would be the first to descend on many awful accidents. He would enter situations that called for on the spot judgment calls. He would act despite the danger involved. He would come to see many shocking and truly terrifying sights. Both Ernie and Esther gave generously in their executions. They had heart felt acceptance towards all kinds of people. Friends, family and strangers would feel their generosity at all times.

Farming was a huge part of Ernie's life. He would tend to the rich soil so he could plant the important seeds. To take Ernie his much needed supper out to the big field was a chore I looked forward to. To see him covered in dusty dirt and smiling made me truly know what his happiness was. Everyone has a special place they call only theirs. Ernie's contentment was found out on those quiet stretched fields of gold. We would watch him with amazement as he would fix and replace parts on machinery. When all was safe we would be allowed to assist him with his capable talent. Any work that might be damaging was being left for Ernie to complete.

We would spend many comforting hours in the shop on the farm. All gathered around the small warm wood burning stove. We would wrap our cold hands around hot chocolate that made even brisk days completely tolerable. Out at the country farm was a place of sheer peace as all troubles of the world would seem to drift away for a short while. I could see why Ernie enjoyed his time out here so much. This soothing place also made mighty explorers out of all of us. You could take a leisurely walk through the spring runoff and find things so intently interesting. Driving the small tractor through thick passages full of weeds and brush was to construct a new passage way. The farm was a place of curiosity to develop ones imagination. The times spent there made me some very happy memories. This same passion for the outdoors still is wrapped up in my being today.

MEMORIES MADE

When I was fourteen or so I would rush home after school to get on this small motorized moped. I would wind up and down the country roads until I came upon the farm that occupied my horse named Blue. He was grey and white and when the colors blended he took on a bluish tone. I would dash to get him saddled up and bridle on. I then would gallop up the dusty road until I met my friend on her stately horse. More of a distance up the windy path took us to another friends place with a huge barn with a great hay loft on their property. The hours would slip away as we would swing on the ropes hanging from the tall loft ceiling. We would land in piles of old straw that would cushion our falls. My days were filled with this awesome fun. My friend went home one day to find out her beautiful horse had been sold by her parents without any warning. She was devastated. Needless to say our days in the loft were over.

On summer weekends when nothing was really planned, me and my twin sister would occupy our friend's house for the duration of the weekend. We reveled in going to her country home. Her place was simply everything ours was not. She had a delightful brook running through their property. A dugout was a ways from the home and was used on occasion for swimming on hot sultry days and nights. We would make rafts from wood and eagerly enter the cold deep water. They also had an entertaining Caboose from a real train in their yard that acted as a play house of sorts. It was always the chosen place to gather and cause mischief. On one day not so different from the rest we decided to try and light the pilot light on the oven so we could bake who knows what. My friend boasted about how this should be dealt with. With such courage she placed her entire head in the dark oven. She struck the match with force and placed the red flame near the place intended. With a very sudden loud thundering boom, the oven was smoking and all the glass windows came crashing in amongst us. My friend slowly backed from the oven and raised her head in shock. She turned around and startled us with her blackened face. She had no facial hair at all. Her eyebrows, eyelashes and hair around her face were gone. She was fine but very scared. We made so much noise that her parents came rushing to the Caboose to see about the commotion.

We made another common visit to this same friend's house on yet another fun filled day. To walk along the brook and just relax and let our minds wander was very calming for us all. We were young teens with much to talk about. So of course these conversations went over so much better with cigarettes. My friend's mom smoked so she was able to sneak one or two often enough that we were never caught. Today was going to be different and difficult. The mother was smart and did notice the smokes were missing. She caught us red handed with smoke exhaling from our mouths and cigarettes in hand. The pissed mom called Esther to see if she could teach us all a valuable lesson. Esther was all for it. She said "what you are going to do will either cure them or kill them". We had to sit in my friend's house on the floor in the middle of the kitchen with buckets nearby for relieving our nausea. We were made to smoke cigarette after nasty cigarette after disgusting cigarette. Well I do think we all became very green with major tobacco breath. I also did use that bucket a time or two. It however never did curb my desire for smoking. I think I just became sneakier about it until I was old enough to do the act in the presence of adults.

The Ponderosa was a special place that we happily would spend our free weekends. This small piece of land was situated on Bear Lake just miles from Grimshaw. The hot muggy days were spent near or on the water. The lake would be an enticing place to venture. To make an unexpected entrance with the tall green reeds swaying in the water always produced the grey worm like Blood Suckers. It never became an enjoyable encounter when these really nasty looking suckers would attach themselves to us like permanent birth marks. We always had salt or matches readily available to attack the disgusting worms. They had a hold of you and would not let go unless you pulled extremely hard on their squishy bodies. They never however limited our joyful activities that were water sports.

We all took our turns patiently learning to water ski. The wood skis would gush us out of the water as if we were determined enough to fly on the lake. Ernie himself could be a bit of a dare devil. When he was gliding on the shimmering water on the strong skis, he would cautiously place the braided rope around his sturdy neck. With all his strength and gull his hands would carefully let go of the rope. He would skillfully balance his weight over the skis and let one of them casually drop. He was now purposely on one ski with a death grip on his neck and no hands for security. He was extremely lucky that nothing seriously ever happened while doing this crazy stunt. One slight mishap could have injured him for life. My own children learned to water ski on the very same wooden water skis that their Grandpa used.

My personal skiing tragedy happened when a huge knot in my tethered rope slipped open while going full speed. I immediately lost control and fell extremely quick and hard on my lower back. I landed with a huge thud on my one remaining ski. I lay in the cool shimmering water aware of my surroundings but not able to verbally talk. The pain in my back was so intense I could not even move slightly. My body only swayed with the ripples of the water as the movement of the oncoming boat came to my rescue. I could hear talking close by but I could not offer any response. With much help I was able to slowly inch my way on to the comfortable boat. With time and stillness, my back pain subsided. Needless to say I never really found the desire to continue with that sport.

My other eventful scare would also happen at the Ponderosa when I was a young teen. Ernie and Esther were on the sturdy boat enjoying the hot lazy day away. I and some friends decided to stay back on land and enjoy the warming fire. Being a knower of all things at my age; the group stupidly put a full glass bottle of our favorite beer in the toasty glowing embers. A close friend had demonstrated at a previous engagement that a glass bottle under direct heat would break clean and smooth all the way around, leaving a perfect cup. We waited for this to magically happen. I became impatient and poked the sizzling hot bottle with a handy stick. At that precise moment of contact with the glass beverage, the bottle exploded. It sent chards of sharp glass in every direction. When it had all finished, I had a direct hit to my bottom lip. The razor edged glass had pierced a complete slice from front to back right through the tender skin. A gash was evident in my forehead and I resembled a bloody villain from a horror movie. My outcome required stitches to both areas of my swollen face. Stupidity was the word for the day.

HOLIDAYS

When the school year would come to a hurried end, we children would be dashing home. We would go on our annual camping vacation for three continuous glorious weeks. This was a ritual every summer. We over the years would test out all makes and models of Recreational Vehicles. The Truck Camper with the big blue bubble windshield on the top bunk was our extreme best. The holiday vehicle of Ernie's choice would be packed with Esther's knowledge of what was to be considered a necessity. Loading the unit for six willing passengers was not an easy task for most. The anticipation of a touring holiday would not come quick enough. Leaving the small town of Grimshaw for a brief while was needed and required. We all tasted the sweet escape to something bigger that would pique our interest away.

Progression of our travels would take us in many directions and various locations. Jasper and Banff became my absolute favorite destination. To this day, I still get captivated by the scenery. When the mountains come into view, you enter another atmosphere. The air becomes cleaner, the tall evergreens are richer and the majestic mountains with snow covered peaks are more fantastic than the last time you saw them. The crystal clear aqua marine lakes take my breath away. I just want to touch it like in a painting before me. We are all here in this very special place under god's watchful eye. Too purposely destruct anything in this true wonderful piece of paradise on earth would be a sin. The precious wild animals like the Bear with claws like nails, Moose with velvet antlers, Mountain Goats with their sure gait and Elk that are the crowd pleaser. These wild animals are present in the vast miles of these protected parks.

Penticton, British Columbia, became our sanctuary for many summers. My eldest sister would take Figure Skating Lessons during the day in a cold arena. My sisters and I swam in the heat of day and leisured in the warm sand.

The lonely winding Forestry Trunk Road was a place of solitude that we entered. There would be no evidence of people present anywhere. The days would pass with no vehicles in sight. We were like new frontiers in an untamed land just waiting to be discovered for the first time. That is how it felt, traveling alone with such quietness. Luckily we never encountered any troubles of any kind along the way. We could have been stuck for days without any assistance. We were very excited when we finished with those rough back roads. The vast Badlands of Drumheller were intoxicatingly interesting. The dry hills with prickly cactus and sage brush made you think about the days of the Dinosaur.

Old Faithful with all its grandness and preciseness was memorizing. The sure force of its gathered hot water holds you in its circle. When she decides to burst, your enthusiasm lets go with shouts and sighs. It becomes so amazing how this natural Geyser has an internal clock for accuracy. This particular place, one must really witness first hand and see it for what it is, remarkable.

Huckleberry Hot springs, with its warm natural water was so soothing. Enjoying its healing ingredients made your body relax and renew.

Butchard Gardens is abundant with gorgeous flowers. The exotic smells take your senses dancing. The colors and patterns make you want this sensation all for your very own. We, as a family over the years were very blessed to have seen wonderful places that I will remember always. Those trips with Ernie and Esther will always stay fresh in my mind. We made memories that were meant to last. Those were the best of times. I will definitely treasure and cherish all the days of my life.

EUROPE

With a wide smile on my fourteen year old face, I was eager to travel to Europe with my sisters and Esther for the six week duration. Esther would have her capable hands full, meeting all four of her daughter's needs. To take on this challenging but rewarding venture was a testament to Esther's character. She would meet this encounter like all others, head first and full of steam. Her efforts would show us that she was a strong individual. She would make us work as a team. This surely would teach us all that Esther's heart was always with her girls. She was healthy and strong and together we could be very united.

Mickey's fish and chips in England were a unique corner diner. They served your meal wrapped in newspaper. The grease from the fried fish was absorbed in the print. This location was the first time I had ever witnessed a man dressed as a woman. Small Alberta towns did not at this time freely show such individualism. It was all very exciting and thrilling to see. My sense of wonder was absorbing these people's traits. This person's identity was so up front and personal. I liked the straight and clear message that was being sent. I am me. This also became a first to see bright colors of hair, like electric blue and neon orange. Such risky trends and straight forwardness seemed worldly. Was I living in a hole somewhere and missed waking up to these new ways. I believe I wanted to be a part of this new age.

In Scotland Esther slept at our relative's home. As it was not large enough for extra occupants, we girls were sent to sleep down the road in a stranger's creepy domicile. Esther was brave to leave us; we were frightened as the owners did not questionably enjoy our company. We did not want Esther to worry as she really had no options, so we kept our fears in check and were thrilled when it was time to move on.

In Holland we discovered a young male was following our moves around the scenic area. This became a little nerve racking and made us aware of probable discomforts. Amsterdam was home to my eldest sister's pen pal. After so many years of communicating through letters, she was finally able to meet her face to face. A pleasant night was coming to an end all too quickly.

Esther and my sister were returning back to our loft in the darkness of night. They were witness to a heart wrenching attack on an individual unaware of his surroundings. The method used to force harm on this person was Brass Knuckles. This very intense large city was showing its violent side.

This same sister also had her priceless wallet stolen. We made our way to the Canadian Embassy for some kind of reassurance. We were just another traveling few that were passing on our information that was heard so often. To us this was a very big deal. To the consultants, we were just more worried partners passing through the lines of continual traffic.

Loading the train in Germany we were met by some of Ernie's family. We did not speak a word of German, so communicating was very difficult. Our hosts were very accepting of us and our language barrier. We settled at their homes and we were made to feel comfortable and at ease. The elderly couple held a Sixteenth Birthday party for my sister. They invited all the neighborhood kids to wish her well. This gesture was so kind and thoughtful. One of the male guests became a pen pal of mine. I would communicate with him over a period of time. Some of the letters I received came in the German dialect. As I could not decode these words, I would get my Grandfather to read them to me in English.

Germany also brought us directly to Ann Franks hiding place behind a wooden book shelf. To actually be there in the same place as she and witness the exact location of her presence was humbling. Being a young girl of fourteen and putting myself in her position made me feel very lucky for the life I live. I felt so saddened for her and the ones she lost. What a remarkable young woman she was. She truly showed bravery in the face of doubt. She along with the others were making their presence known with education from her words written. Those undeniable moments of discovering places with Esther, made me extremely proud of her.

HAWAII

Hawaii was our next destination for hot sunny days and adventurous nights. Only Esther and the twins were escaping this time. The beaches were perfect and inviting with sand so soft and warm. Our days of leisure were spent lathering ourselves with just the right amount of tanning oil juices. The excursions were made with enthusiastic minds set on learning interesting facts. This introduced us to many places that were full of Hawaiian culture. The new faces we would search on these constant tours were just like us, looking for the differences in life and reveling in the contrast from our own.

Our nights seemed to drift towards a peculiar but fantastic local county bar. The flavor of patrons would be considered the kind that Naval Bases were made of. There was nothing but a generous amount of men and women occupying the dusty floor. They all made their way here to this spot from their working ships in port. This particular group of people surly needed no encouragement to show off their dancing skills. The country music with a twang was made for two stepping. The line dances were perfected on the dance floor with precision. These talented men and women where completing these line dances singular. This was an absolutely new take for me on how country dancing should go. I had no choice but to join in and be part of this spectacle that was full of energy and exuded such happiness. The sweat in the air was almost a pleasant one. We would never have this chance again probably to dance among these men and women that deserved so much gratitude from their country. To have this much camaraderie in one place left me feeling whole and satisfied. Our continued laughter and high spirits made us all feel a part of something very unique. Esther would get to witness our laughter and smiles of glee. Every night possible we would make our way to this bar that was starting to place a stamp on our hearts.

One night so like the others, a situation transpired when a persistent man would badger me incisively. To my ecstatic relief a perfect gentleman was placed right behind me. He could see that I required immediate assistance. I gladly and graciously accepted his help with making a truce known. This kind man realized we were tourists. He extended his kindness once more with inviting us to visit him on the USS Kitty Hawk. This ship was known as a gem among all others. He was stationed in port. Esther's gypsy side took over and without a doubt we were at the harbor the next day. What was so intriguing to me was that as a Canadian, I really never even knew these massive ships were in existence. I for sure never new one of these water vessels could carry and land planes and jets on their deck. The sheer size of these ships was amazing. What a thrill it was to be shown the innards of this grand floating dwelling. We had front row seats to every inch of that ship. We truly had a memorable day that we would never forget. I also made a dear friend for life that day. His physical presence cannot be seen, as the distance is too huge a barrier. As I am a Canadian living in Alberta and he a US citizen residing in Florida. We have conversed with each other for over thirty years now. His friendship is very important and true to me. Maybe we will meet again but if not the memories never fade.

My special friend from Hawaii did however mention that one day he would show up unexpectedly in Grimshaw unannounced. He was true to his word. He along with another male friend actually pulled up to Ernie's car dealership in a black shiny truck. His prediction had come to life. Two years from our meeting, he had driven the distance to make an epic reunion a classic. We were all in amazement with their presence. It was truly a shock for me to see him face to face in my home town. Nothing was planned in advance as their arrival was unexpected. As autumn was upon us, Ernie would take the two men harvesting. Riding in the combine was a new adventure for them. The Peace River Hills were a beautiful sight with the red and golden leaves. A boat ride down the Mighty Peace River was an exciting one. The wonderment of it all was ours to give. The sharing we were showing made me very grateful to my family for extending their joy onto them. Our time together was a thoughtful gesture on their part. I at this time in my life had a boyfriend I adored. He was so sweet as to not get offended by their presence. They had traveled the many long miles for a simple girl. I had nothing to give in return, but my willingness to show them a tiny fragment of my existence.

GRIMSHAW/BERWYN GRADUATION

The year I graduated was full of lasting magical memorable times. 1981 was the year I turned eighteen. My graduation was set for Friday night. On Thursday a group of us were at the spot that would host our Grad party for Friday evening. We were antsy to get the festivities started. A bunch of us were gathered around the enormous fire pit. One of the eager boys decided that the fire would start quicker if some gasoline was poured over the dry exposed wood. I could tell that this act was not going to go according to his plan. Many of us backed away from the pit knowing a disaster was imminent. Sure enough the splintered wood caught fire so quickly that the blaze became an instant inferno. One of my fellow class mates was standing too close and the material on his arm caught on fire. He was so alarmed that he was running and falling trying to buff out the flames. Some intelligent guys that had their smarts about them took off their jean jackets and tried to snuff out the flames as best they could. The young guy in distress hit the ground one more time not knowing what direction the fire pit was in. He rolled so close to the embers that he was engulfed once more. This time his charred arm was smothered successfully. In all the grad pictures this poor fellow has a bandage around his swollen aching arm.

My grad day came and went. It was what was to be expected. I had my boyfriend of three years near my side. My parents were proud of me. I was thrilled that school was done at last after thirteen years. It is what went on the next day being Saturday night that still can make me shake and my voice quiver.

In grade nine, the small town of Berwyn were bussing their students to Grimshaw High to complete the rest of their senior courses. My new boyfriend happened to be one of these new students. His cousin started seeing my best friend at the time. All four of us spent much time together. These were special times spent with close friends. I continued to date my boyfriend right into my twelfth year of school. Grimshaw's Grad was completed. Some of us were still functioning from the night before. We were still ready to party on. The thought came to us that we needed to celebrate with the Berwyn Grads at their bash. We knew my boyfriend's cousin would be there so we felt sure to be welcomed. We had become close and made lasting friendships with many of the Berwyn kids as they had spent much time in Grimshaw. Four of us piled into my friends black pickup truck. There was myself, my girlfriend and two other boys. We arrived at this party that was unlike any other. There was immediate chaos all around. The two males that were stationed with us vacated the truck instantly. We were left by the vehicle with terror in our eyes. The first thing that registered to me was that a guy was getting a wine bottle smashed over the center of his head. I was confused by all the needless action taking place around us. I could see the big bonfire in the near distance.

Several people were surrounding it. My girlfriend and I were not close really to anything but in the middle of everything. My boyfriend's cousin came by us aimlessly in complete and utter shock. He was showing us the hole someone had bitten into his fore arm. He was full of intense anger and frustration. He left us in a hurry. Our two male friends that came with us in the truck showed up gasping for air. Before we could say, "what the hell is going on here" they vanished again. Some guys were here and they all had their shirts off for some reason. They seemed to belong together, like a gang. The strange fellows were completely sober, which was a little peculiar for a Grad party. I finally had realized who these people were. A family of boys from Peace River with a bad reputation. They were not well liked in Grimshaw or Berwyn. They had purposely shown up later in the evening when most people were already intoxicated. They took full advantage of that situation. They were ready to cause some uncontrollable damage on certain people. They had a plan in effect and were scouting out the individuals that they wanted to fight with. Then it switched into hurting whomever happened to be in there way. We were still just standing by the truck in awe of what was happening around us. Our confused eyes were now directed to the fire pit. People were being herded into the earth at the fires edge by a vehicle. Our registered warnings took over our senses. My strong girlfriend grabbed me by the scruff of the neck and literally threw me inside the black awaiting truck. We locked the doors and were so nervous. Where were our friends? Finally the boys showed up. Someone needed to contact the police and give them directions to the party. This gathering had turned into a violent rampage. The electrified boys took their places in the truck. We sped to the nearest farm house and called for help. (No cell phones invented yet) We met the Police in Berwyn. We would show them the way back out to the hell that was waiting. As we arrived the sky was starting to clear and brighten up as early morning was upon us. The sight that greeted us was sickening. A man lay in the back of a truck with two broken legs. He was there just like us to celebrate with friends. The fire pit contained all the glass from broken beer bottles. An unwilling victim entered this disaster area and was cut severely. He was in need of medical care like so many others out there. Many were on their way to the small Berwyn hospital. We took the time to glance around the party area now. It was becoming light out we had sadness in our eyes. Then what we saw made us raw with fury. The Peace River boys were still there gloating and full of pride. It was not hard to figure out who the perpetrators were. They were prancing around with bare chests. The presence of the police did not bother them at all. They had to of seen the damage they had done to various people. Many of them were still there badly hurt. We definitely had enough and again maneuvered back to the hospital. One of my male friends started to walk over to us after being attended to.

One of the instigators glared at him and said "I know who you are". After all had been done I finally appeared at home around six a.m. I dashed with scared determination to my twin sister's room to voice the craziness that had just gone on. Ernie came rushing into the room to make sure I was ok. Morning coffee had already gotten the news around that a night of celebration turned into a night of total destruction.

After all the madness was over I went back to work at the Bakery in Peace River. Often I would cross paths with these sketchy Peace River guys. I knew they recognized me. It always sent shivers up my spine. I then changed jobs and started working at the Court House in Peace River. When this all went to trial I often would have to enter the Court room. My nerves would catch up to me as soon as the door would inch open. I would see these short stout guys turn my way. Talking about this even now and writing about it still gets me worked up. The Ice Road Trucker and I were both at that Berwyn Grad Party. His brother was my good friend. His cousin was my boyfriend at the time. He writes about this same party in his book, The King of the Road. The Grad to end all Grads made news in the Alberta Report. It was not long after that dry Grads and supervised Grads were put into play.

TRIAL CAMPING RUN

With two babies in tow, my husband and I were willing to go the distance to make new tales of our own. We were anxious, ready and willing to advance to survival Camping 101 with our son and daughter. We rushed to provide all the necessities we would require. My son was a mere three weeks old and my sweet daughter was one and a half. We crammed our very small round Scamper trailer to the max. This was to be our trial run camping close to home. If we could master this, we could take on a bigger project. We could possibly try to deliver us all to Shaw's Point in one piece. I was relieved that my post pregnancy body was not producing any more enriched milk. The prescribed dry up pills were working fantastically. My babies so close in age were both on bottles with my encouragement. My beautiful daughter of sixteen months was in the process of becoming zippy cups coinsure. It was all working perfectly with both of them cooperating with the drinking situation. In the middle of the dark restless night I woke up with extreme anxiety. I stated to my husband that something felt extremely wrong with my breasts. Over the course of hours, they had become completely engorged with milk. I was ready to burst with an explosion of white rich milk everywhere. I wanted so desperately to have my eager son suckle to relieve this problem. He had never breast fed but was very ready. I was content with him on the bottle and he also seemed adequately nourished. With my husband working long hours, this just was not going to be an option. With great discomfort, we took my stretchy bra and tightened it like a corset around my extra-large boobs. The pain subsided within a couple of days. Other than the sleepless nights the trip succeeded without further incidents. Future trips could be seen on the horizon.

CAMPING RITUALS

The Haas Clan started occupying Shaw's Point Resort by High Prairie in and around 1990. We would mostly gather at the resort during the July long weekend. The girls and their families along with Ernie and Esther have been drifting and congregating there for twenty five years or more. We have spent thousands of our dollars keeping the point prosperous and functional along with other park attendants. When times have been tough on the consumer we have continued to make Shaw's Point our home away from home. We faithfully pull up our convoy and find pleasure in our short or lengthy stays. There was only one much needed marina in the beginning. The shower room was used plenty. It was placed at the back of the main office by the entrance where the world sized fish is in sight. There are now two well-equipped marinas with pontoon rentals and gas for your recreational and fishing boats. Gladly they installed up to date showers and urinals. The old wooden outhouses still remain, but now we are not forced to visit them. A full meal restaurant is situated overlooking the second marina. Favorable ice cream and tasty pie is served warm. This is the best place to witness the catches of the day. The fish cleaning stations are always occupied. Mini Golf keeps the swarm of children occupied for hours. Our own kids spent many a day exercising their limbs at the pink plastic playground. The beach would be covered with sun worshippers with the hot rays of summer. The young and old enjoy the cool water and shady trees. The lots for sale and rent have increased by bounds. We literally have put our mark on every inch of this property. We have weathered through windblown days. Our tiny tin can trailers would became sweat lodges at night. We spent soaked days and nights trapped behind tarps that could not relieve you from the shuddering cold. The dry, dusty days of wind would cause fire bans. The moist dewy rain would splurge on the flooding. Drunken nights of silliness was not often but could be blamed away with the longevity of the night. Minor emergencies were tended too through the years. We have celebrated Happy Birthdays and mile stone Anniversaries. We are always planning for the next excursion out to Shaw's Point.

If you were to ask the grandchildren of Ernie and Esther what was their one favorite time at Shaw's Point, they would without hesitation say the awesome fishing. Every night it became a ritual to rent a large pontoon. The perfect time to stroll out of the busy marina was when the sunlight was starting to fade away. You were in direct line with the slow moving light. The reflection off the still water was blinding to the naked eye. If the dandelion fuzz was abundant and just skimming the water's surface, the calm ripples were perfect for this talented sport. Spitz in one hand and fish scales on the other meant for a good catch. Slippery minnows, long slimy leeches and the black of diamonds head were the bait of choice. With years of experience behind us we have all been introduced to the pink, yellow and black jig heads made of rubbery material. With just a minnow and hook on the end of the pole to master the talented craft of fishing. The tackle boxes were supplied with various hooks and showed off with pride. Each person would try to demonstrate their unique pick of tackle and send the line to the depths beneath. The reels would be exercised and sent out with its best deliverance. The lines would be infested with the constant nibbles of the unaware fish. The lines were so quick with takers that it was a baiting frenzy on board. Being back on land meant the gutting station was the next step in preparation for a feast. The evening tantalized your taste buds with fish fried to perfection. The recipes are the same. Simple is best when frying fish. Green onion and Shake n Bake are used as batter for the flavor which urges you to taste the undeniable succulent fish. After the evening of filling our bellies it was time for a warm fire and great company. Caramelized marshmallows have also become a Haas favorite. We still return to this vacation spot every year when possible. With new additions to the family I greatly hope that this tradition will continue.

REWARDS OF HARD WORK

Esther and Ernie both came from humbling backgrounds. What they had in material, they had worked extremely hard for. They had no hand outs and strived to acquire possessions they never were fortunate to have growing up. I believe that their creative desires built a path for them. Doors opened to those who knew how to cherish and relish in the opportunities that came before them. They never took their forth comings for granted. You can be given all on a silver platter but it can lose its shine very quickly if not properly cared for. To finally accumulate property, meant to have a future to smile at. Ernie and Esther made the simple things seem special. To see a morning sunrise meant another day of blessings. To conquer another years battles and forge ahead was gratifying. When seedlings would force through the hard winterized ground, spring would be full of new challenges to take on. Frozen rivers and lakes would melt away and make room for the Canadian Geese that were returning home. Babies of the earth are welcomed to a new world of wonder. To give someone a simple smile or a friendly nod could change the outcome of someone's day. To give your assistance was an unselfish act and required nothing in return. These acts of kindness would be acted upon instinctively. Hopefully these teachings are absorbed into the next generation's way of thinking. Maybe the world will survive if taught in time.

ESTHER'S CHALLENGES

Esther's head would heal drastically since her major surgery. This meant it was definitely time to complete the task of correcting her double vision. Ten months post her serious operation, on October Eighth, 1998 at twelve thirty p.m. her Doctor was successful in the procedure. Esther would reluctantly have to wear a large bandage on her face for a period of time. Her right eye would be blurry and sore. Eye drops were prescribed and used properly. With time her vision would return back to normal.

Esther would be administered into the Grimshaw Hospital on November Twenty Fourth, 1998. She was experiencing extreme pain in her legs and back. The severe aches were stronger than the usual. The doctor's suggestion was to adhere to strong Morphine. The intolerable pain was subsided when the powerful medicine was used. It would however make Esther nauseated for the duration of her stay. The Morphine was successful and did achieve at taking away the soreness. She was finally able to get this situation under control and be back at home shortly.

HEART ATTACK #1

One and half years had passed since Esther's major surgery. Ernie entered his welcoming home at eleven thirty a.m. on April Twenty Third, 1999 looking terrible with an indescribable pain in his tight chest. Ernie had made an urgent stop at the Doctor's office; they stated he should proceed to the hospital immediately. Ernie then placed himself cautiously into his Chevy truck. Priority was given to his place of employment first. He realized that his desk had plenty of cash and cheques in his private drawer. Once those were collected then he could proceed. He quickly had to drop off Esther's important Morphine prescription. He required those necessities to get placed at home first. He then paced himself to the hospital. The dread his body was now feeling was calling his name from the walls of the emergency room. Ernie staggered to the main entrance door of the small hospital. He practically fell in the glassed doorway. A neighbor friend was following behind him and steadied his pace. Ernie was indeed having a massive heart attack. Ernie's second eldest daughter left her job and came immediately to tend to Ernie. She arrived to the hospital to be by his painful side. One of Ernie's twin daughters carefully and mindfully picked up Esther at home. They quickly drove to the nearby entrance. Ernie was a very serious case. He was dutifully placed in the Air Ambulance to Grande Prairie Hospital. This location was an hour and a half away. Ernie would have his second daughter as a passenger on the rough ride to Grande Prairie. She would not sway from Ernie's side until late in the evening. She then with hesitation left for the remainder of the night to a nearby hotel. As daylight approached, Esther followed through to Grand Prairie the next day. Her other daughters would make Esther's approach to Ernie a safe one. My husband and I would make the long drive from Westlock to see Ernie personally. This round trip would take fourteen hours. The journey was tiring and mentally challenging. We gathered up our strength and entered the room where Ernie was positioned. He was hooked up to multiple machines. As soon as I saw him under these foreign conditions I started to tear up. He was so tired and just totally exhausted. He had been through so much chaos already. Now his heart would become a huge deterrent in his daily living.

Ernie would with focus have to impress the Doctors with his strength. The stress tests would be measured and their findings would determine his being released. He had sufficiently finished his series of tests. On Wednesday the twenty eighth of April at 3:30 p.m. he had passed enough to qualify for a release and was eager to get back to Grimshaw. Esther was very surprised that Ernie was on his way back home from the Grande Prairie Hospital so soon. Upon Ernie's arrival he immediately fell into boss mode and required all of his important keys. An impaired grim stare reluctantly showed on Esther's face.

She had no recollection as to the whereabouts of Ernie's precious metal. They both searched the big house for several hours with no success. Finally the eldest daughter had a flash and remembered the tagged keys were placed in the small entrance closet for safe keeping. Esther said with a grunt, "how the hell could I forget that, as it was so very important."

ESTHER'S SCHOOL REUNION

Esther was looking forward to her Berwyn School Reunion, The Class of 1959. This was an event Esther was longing to attend. The Wine and Cheese party was held on the second of June to commence the official start of the Berwyn Reunion. A very dear friend of Esther's made a special appearance at this function. The day was made perfect with the closeness they got to share for the duration of the day. Esther had commented on how everyone looked so young in class pictures back then. She noticed that the majority of the guests all had developed some graying hair, increased their weight and were wearing glasses. Time had a way of making youthful bodies decline with age. Esther had coped with the exercises of the day extremely well. She digested two extra pain pills which relaxed her to enjoy the festivities. Esther was impressed with the meal as her appetite was back to normal. They arrived home that evening at eleven p.m., drained from all the activities. She was so ecstatic that the day had glided as smoothly as she had hoped for.

Esther was up to the challenge of continuing on with the gathering, as her body was cooperating thankfully. She would make the extra effort to engage with her old friends. The Alley Cat Skipping Rope Team did all their tricks necessary for the captive audience. Even an old boyfriend made a special attempt to be courteous. They followed up by reminiscing about parties held at his parent's house in the days back when. Esther was enjoying all of it and captivated by the wonderful company. Some strangers entered as it was also a reunion for Ernie's grade and up. This however was not a problem and did not matter to Esther. She could communicate with anyone and adapt to the current conversation. She noticed that only two of the many attendees walked with visible canes such as her. The evening was memorable and Esther was thrilled that she had participated in the fun. Ernie practically had to force Esther to leave, as midnight was upon them. The Banquet, Entertainment and long overdue conversation with friends made for an extremely pleasurable evening.

Five consecutive days with relativity no pain was great news for Esther. This was a rare occurrence for her. The day just continued to get better. Her thoughtful sisters which she didn't get to see often had managed a visit in the late afternoon and left beautiful flowers. The pungent smell drifting from the gorgeous bouquet needed to evaporate some. They were placed outside so they could absorb the pure air. Esther just could not tolerate the fragrance the buds and blossoms were exuding. Her day was complete with more company. Ernie's only brother and his traveling companion, his wife, were next for visiting. They were making their annual trip from Ontario. The couples chatted before the nights end. Esther always looked forward to their visits as her sister-in-law was a dear friend.

ERNIE'S BROKEN WRIST

Fourteen months after Esther's operation, Ernie had another accident. Esther was exiting the front door to the house. She wanted to voice to Ernie her concern. She didn't like the fact that he was steadying himself on the top step of the metal ladder. Just as her mind registered the thought, Esther heard a loud abrasive crashing sound. Ernie had lost his balance and fell to the hard ground. His wrist had lodged its self in between the metal steps on his way to connecting with the earth. Ernie was encouraged by his sudden pain to inch his way to the house entrance. His wounded hand was hanging strangely. Ernie's words came out in distorted fashion. He absolutely was headed to the Grimshaw Hospital with needful urgency. Ernie was quite positive that his injured wrist or hand was most likely broken. Ernie's twin daughter met him at the emergency entrance. Ernie was returned back home with his pride a little tarnished and his extremely sore wrist bandaged in a cast. That restless long lasting dark night, Ernie had severe pain and slept very poorly. With Esther not being capable of too much extra physically, her mental support was beneficial. Ernie had been preparing the meals for them both. Now Esther was going to have to step in and replace that duty. The girls would once again pitch in and help. They would manage to keep both Ernie and Esther progressing in a positive way. It was suggested by the experts that Ernie should surrender two months off work. His wrist required time to heal properly. That Sunday the First of August, Ernie was to have his wrist rewrapped in a preferred new cast. The original position was not placed correctly. For maximum and beneficial use it would be set again. Ernie was happily induced with pain medicine. The doctor basically took his painfully swollen wrist and manipulated it to the proper setting. Even with Ernie under sedation I could still grasp that he felt the intense sensation of hurt. His face would contort into features that were showing signs of agony. Ernie would have a date set to see a specialist in Grande Prairie on the Tenth of August. The holiday that they both had looked so forward to was on hold for the time being.

Ernie was off to complete his annual tarring the roof on his main street building in Grimshaw. This structure was old and always needed tending too. This particular task would easily take up his whole weekend. This was always done with only him in attendance. This job was supervised only by one man, and his name was Ernie. To hand this dirty job over to a qualified individual was not heard of. Even with his wrist in a bothersome cast, Ernie was game to finish this ritual his way. He would not surrender until his shift was over. We would catch a glimpse of him on the roof and wish we could partner him. You just can't teach a stubborn mind any different.

When September Eighth of 1999 came upon us, Ernie was relieved that his nuisance of a cast was coming off without delay. Esther's mind was full of worry though.

Ernie was in terrible pain. His huge hand was extremely pale white and his swollen arm was hurting with every movement made. Due to his lack of usage, his wrist was still mending and would take time to properly heal as thought. His other functioning arm was now quite sore as he had been over compensating for his immobile arm for quite some time.

ESTHER'S PLEASURES

Esther was a history buff follower and enjoyed this form of writing from an early age. She loved to read about distant foreign places and times in the long ago past. Reading about such things took up a lot of her unoccupied time. We however did not seem to share her enthusiasm for affairs not current and not pertaining to the present. Esther was translating a family history story. It was about our relatives from the Jaffrey clan. We were not purposely showing any real interest in her passion and kept interrupting her train of thought. Esther became upset and frustrated with us. She thought we were being absolutely rude for muttering laughter and talking under our breaths engaged in small talk through her conversation. Finally Esther conveyed her outrage and Ernie looked embarrassed. Esther cried somewhat after her explosion of words and translated how she felt. "I feel invisible sometimes. Ernie really does try to focus and listens to my ramblings and I fall apart with bursts of crying. I am actually rather mad and just get completely frustrated; I can't do what I want." Esther continued to force out her explanation, "You are all trying really hard to understand. I know it frazzles you to see me, as I am. It is a hell of a thing."

My twin sister was at Esther's giving her assistance so graciously. She was aiding Esther with her extremely large collection of family pictures. Pacing through all the memories she was seeing before her, was like reliving the act all over. The faces of the elderly, young and infant would make her emotions surface. The small tears would start to discard and roll softly down her cheeks. She really tried to maintain and control her composure as her two granddaughters were also helping with the task at hand. Esther had not taken her anti-anxiety pill for the day on purpose. She wanted to find out just how she would really truly feel without the interruption of the strong medication in her system. Every time Esther would eat she would have a multitude of different waves of pain. Esther's aching was persistent and common on a daily basis. She would experience surges of acute pain through her whole charged body. The worst kind of cruelty was when this in tolerable force of agony went straight for the damaged head. Esther would have little pain on the left side of her being. The Tumor was located on the left side of her spinal cord and skull. Due to the placing, Esther would then experience most of her trauma on the opposite, being the right side of her body.

Esther would have a ritual when it came to getting ready for her night of slumber. This I believe was also her way of relaxing herself and putting her surroundings at bay for a while. She could not control most things in her life anymore but this one important issue was hers alone to master. This practice she completed every evening no matter what. She would wash her tired beautiful face. Then she would apply a generous amount of Nivea cream to her barely wrinkled face. Vaseline would be smeared and spread under her eyes. Her face was virtually flawless to the signs of aging. She had done this routine most of her adult life. Her toes were then cleaned individually. Vaseline Lotion would then be smeared onto her baby soft feet. Her bright white teeth were cleaned with brushing and flossing. This rite of passage she felt was a gift and not a hindrance. She treasured this quiet time. She certainly had the most glowing skin and perfect touchable feet that a lady could ever wish for. The last thing before the lights went out was to administer one ounce of laxative and two pain pills.

FORTY YEARS TOGETHER

Ernie and Esther's Fortieth Anniversary was arriving soon on September Twenty Sixth. We wanted to celebrate with something special. We put forth notices to Esther's brothers and sisters. Each was instructed to compile a twelve inch by twelve inch piece of material. Each square was to reflect their individuality. This material could be any type decorated to their specific liking. The family would in return forward this material back to us. Then the pieces were all collected and sewn together to make a beautiful, colorful and unique quilt. Esther and Ernie would be able to reflect on each person's imagination through the loving pieces that were done so with care and thoughtfulness. What was also special about that glorious day was that Ernie's brother and sister in law arrived from Ontario. We were all fortunate to spend this time with them. A delicious homemade supper was included in the evening at their daughter's house. She has become an expert at cooking and enjoys the challenge. We devour her tasty morsels with vigor. The evening was enjoyed by all. Ernie and Esther were so surprised with the beautiful gift. The quilt that was made for them was a perfect way to show our love and affection.

A PROMISE MADE

Having made a solid promise to Esther about quitting smoking was weighing on my mind heavily. I was struggling with the fact that two years had passed and I was still blowing smoke, literally. Her sentence of two to five years of survival was arriving now. She positively just had to see me quit this nasty habit before her death. I would not be able to live with the disgrace of breaking an oath. With every fiber of my being this huge obstacle had to be met head on. I was ready to sell my soul to the devil if I had to. Today I was becoming a nonsmoker. This meant many things would become off limits. I had to purposely not put myself into situations that would tempt me. I was no different than any other person with an addiction. An Alcoholic doesn't go to a bar, gambler to a casino, junky to a dealer and a smoker will find a way to inhale that toxic grey matter any way possible. There was times when my husband and I did not mesh to good together when I first quit. He would want to go socialize at a local function or to a close tavern for the evening. I would have to fight with the good and bad devil in my head. Of course I wanted to go participate in the gathering but that also would mean the temptation of failure. This would put me in many situations of having to defend myself with my husband, family and friends. I will honestly say that I became a nasty little bitch to live with.

I might have given in to the desire one night about

three months into my living clean without cigarettes. I was sitting around the perfect campfire that had me mesmerized at Shaw's Point. My brother in law and I were the last of the crew to still be drinking heavily into the night. Since it was just us, we decided in our drunken haze to go visit other campers still forging ahead at this late hour. The usual busy camp ground was still and peaceful except for the likes of us. I completely and utterly lost my lack of judgment. My senses were so mixed up that I lit a delightful smoke. I rather enjoyed it at that moment. Immediately after indulging in that now rancid cigarette, I had a sudden wave of nausea came over me. My head was circling and my stomach was flopping every which way. This awful sensation brought me to my knees with sickness. I vomited in the tiny trailer bathroom. All night long I was forced to surrender myself to the urinal until six a.m. That gross sensation of wooziness never left me until well into the next day. Now if I ever have the itch to fantasize about a cigarette, I think of that long drawn out night of hung over hell.

The actual act of smoking was not too hard to give up. It was the socializing with your peers that was hard to let go of. You had this habit that was common among you all. You seemed to belong in the circle, no matter who was present. This sense of kinship was uniform wherever you lit up. My twin sister and my husband would gather by an open window and strategically force the mixed air out as not to bother me. I finally said, "please come and sit with me and have the damn thing right here." I felt excluded in my own home. This sense of abandonment could have brought me right back to inhaling poison again. It was a true measure of my willingness to do what I had promised Esther that made me succeed. My husband would join the nonsmoking league about six years after me. We were now gladly both committed to being nonsmokers. Esther did get to see me accomplish this most difficult task. My sacrifices were minor compared to hers. Esther was tackling her vices every day. Thanks for the push Esther.

ONE FINGER

Ernie had been traveling the route to Sulphur Lake Road for numerous years. Ernie was familiar with most of the roads, trails, cut lines and creeks on this piece of bumpy road. It was a peaceful place for him and others to go to escape the reality of our lives. The smell of evergreens, wet moss and freshly cut wood was always pleasing to the senses. Ernie would stock his reliable truck with hot cocoa and some canned wieners and beans, off to the bush he would travel. He would shoot a rather simple partridge if it happened to cross his path. Ernie mostly went to clear his mind and soul. He would get rejuvenated for the long week ahead. Taking care of Esther could be challenging and rewarding. This particular journey to Sulphur was like so many before. He got up early with the singing birds. He traveled alone for one and a half hours with his inner thoughts. He navigated his way to a secluded cut line. He was foraging wood for the comforting fireplace and outside yard fire pit. He prepared his chainsaw with a massive pull on the cord. The rumbling sound from the trusty saw could be heard for miles. Ernie continued to put forth his strength to push the jagged teeth of the saw through the old knotty wood. His pile of birch wood was gathered and adding in height. This task was on its way well to being finished. Suddenly the saw skipped and bounced on a knot in the hard wood. With Ernie being slightly relaxed, the dangerous saw hit down to where his left hand was balancing the remaining piece of birch. The many teeth from the sharp edged saw had landed on the second finger of his hand. His protective skin and meaty tissue were tore all up and completely off the bone except for a splinter of skin. Ernie stared at the sight of his blood, skin, and tendons and liquid that was running from his mangled finger. Just as he was assessing the situation, a family friend slowed his vehicle to an idling position and said, "Hello." Ernie never asked for assistance, and his friend drove away down the dusty trail. Ernie wrapped his badly swollen finger with the rest of his attached member with some cloth he had handy. With all of Ernie's belongings stationed back in the truck, he methodically headed off to the Grimshaw Hospital. The agonizing pulse in his finger became intrudingly more persistent.

The non-resembling finger was stitched together with the only real purpose of being attached. The finger would not be mobile or have any usage. Ernie could still say he had five fingers on each hand, even though one of them was useless.

ESTHER'S PARENTS

Esther and her sister would have many conversations over the years about her childhood. She was told that most decisions were made without her consent. The siblings of Esther placed her where they thought were the suitable homes. Esther was grown now and had her own residence in Grimshaw. Grimshaw was the closest town to Peace River. With that being said she was to be the most capable aid for her mother. Esther's mom was diseased with polio. At that period of time there was no establishment for special cased people like Esther's mother. The Auxiliary Hospital in Peace River was a Long Term Facility that had just finished being built. Esther's brother-in-law was on the hospital board. Esther brought it forward that this establishment could be just the place for her mother. Esther's mother was physically challenged. She also had an intricate colostomy. This attachment was nerve racking for the family. Fortunately Esther's mother was accepted to be a permanent patient. Esther and her family were torn with the decision to make it a reality. She would be a distance for the majority of her family. She could hardly walk and needed so much care. For everyone's mental stability, she became one of the first patients to be attending the hospital on a permanent basis. She was probably about sixty three years old when she became a member. She still crafted with her hands. She spent much time with her delicate embroidering work. She continued on with her enjoyable writing. At the age of seventy three she had her Kidney removed that was not functioning properly. At seventy eight she survived a serious stroke and lost her mobility on her right side. She could barely talk and make simple conversation. She however did recover quite well with time. She lived to be a remarkable eighty years old.

Esther's dad was making a living running the family farm. His trapping the cut lines and using the Lumber Mill when he could also made way for earnings. He was slipping away from Stomach Cancer. He departed our world and joined the next, at the age of fifty six.

Esther had a wonderful visit with her sister in August of 2000. She was able to pass on important information. Matters were discussed that had been buried for way to long. She was relieved to talk about family issues in private.

Esther had in years past requested funds from her mother's estate. She was entitled to it legally. Her father's will was issued to protect his wife. It was also to guardian his two youngest children, which happened to be Esther and her little brother. The two little ones were so small and young and could not properly take care of themselves. Her father's land could not be sold until his youngest son turned twenty one. But then her father died and his estate became his wife's. The lands in question now could not be sold until her mother's passing at the age of eighty. Esther inherited her mother's funds from her estate as she was the youngest living child. The little brother was entitled to his father's share. This brother then died and the funds were now transferred to his mother's estate. So with both parents deceased and her little brother departed, all the estate funds went to Esther as she was still the youngest child surviving. This very small fortune would cause great concern for Esther. The small amount of money inherited paid for funeral expenses, grave stone and outstanding bills. The left over funds, Esther graciously used to get copies of old prints made for her sisters and brothers.

HEART ATTACK #2

Ernie had just spent the last two agonizing days in the Intensive Care Unit in Peace River. He had suffered another severe Heart Attack. Ernie would be flown in the Air Ambulance. My eldest sister would join him in the chopper from Peace River to Edmonton. My husband and I would immediately travel from Bonnyville to the Royal Alec Hospital in the city. We would gather forces upon our arrival. We galloped through the long stretched hallways. With purpose we finally emerged to the correct section. My body was commanding me to slow down for a brief moment to catch my breath. This was a different hospital to navigate in. We quietly pulled open the sliding curtain to access the small surrounding area by Ernie's metal single bed. He lay under a crisp clean white linen sheet. All his belongings were placed in a large brown paper bag. The bag was labeled with his name so it would not be misplaced. There were many other patient's laying on beds the same. Ernie was in extreme pain in his lower legs as his Gout was prominent. His feet were swollen and puffy with redness. The nurses had administered a large amount of drugs. The continued pain that he was coping with now became somewhat tolerable with the medication.

We would spend hours sitting restlessly all day by his bedside so Ernie was not alone. When he would fall asleep slightly we would go pace the hallways. This was a way to cope and continue to be strong for him. All the patient's had been operated on and came back for recovery. Ernie was still to be accessed. As the morning turned into night, Ernie was finally placed in a room in another section of the hospital for the evening. Tomorrow was another day full of questions to be answered and acted on. Today and the day before were occupied with lengthy hours. My husband had gone back to Bonnyville. My sister and I would be here until we were required no more. Our practice was to make sure that Ernie was under sedation before we left for some needed sleep and a wholesome meal at our nearby hotel.

With another night upon us, we really debated if we should leave Ernie. We were prepared to sleep on the couches in the nearby waiting room. Our worry was that he would become coherent and become confused and startled. We plainly just did not want him to wake up and not have his bearings about him. He was a big man but to us at this moment he was so fragile and weak.

We left due to the fact that the nurses would surely call should anything pressing happen. Our hotel was literally only five minutes away. We desperately required some space. To function and navigate the next couple of days, we replenished with caffeine and chocolate. We were prepared and equipped with our new set of nerves. It was imperative that we tackle this new day with extra energy. His well-being was our first priority. Our minimal sleep was short and off to the hospital we merged. We should have listened to our intuition. Ernie had a very sleepless night indeed. Sometime through Ernie's haze, he woke up and was not fully balanced. Through his blurred fog he noticed he had the IV inserted into his arm. Without a moment's hesitation or complete thought he pulled the attached needle from his arm. The IV insert was leaking his bodily fluids. Ernie then made his way over to his nearest roommate. He woke him up by placing himself on the edge of the small bed. Ernie then started a pleasant conversation with his neighbor. Ernie was leaving a deep red trail of blood behind him. He was not aware or even cared to notice that he was leaving a disturbing mess. This gentle man was so kind to mask his startled reaction with calm and patience. He quietly and carefully called the nurses for some assistance. My sister and I felt so guilty for not staying with Ernie. We felt complete and utter compassion for this stranger that showed much caring towards a helpless man in need. Ernie would continue his stay and spend more time at the Royal Alec. The wise and experienced doctors were determining what the best course of action was. At first Open Heart Surgery was discussed, he would be transported over to the University of Alberta Hospital in Edmonton. As we were coming to terms with the situation, Esther was at home trying to be self-sufficient without Ernie's aid. As in a usual crisis like this, some of the children would adhere to Ernie and some would stay with Esther and her worries. With further deliberation, the doctors chose to forgo the Open

Heart Surgery. His best chance of survival at this point was not to put any undue stress on him. Ernie might make it through the surgery but the recuperation time might be to damaging. Ernie was not in the best of mental or physical shape, to continue home and heal properly. The doctors decided to clear Ernie's ninety eight per cent blocked arteries with stints instead. The three veins were cleared and Ernie just had a small incision to take care of.

He would of course have to not drive or do any kind of strenuous activities. These orders were hard for a man of men to live with. He would have stressful times no matter what. It was going to be a challenge to heal when he knew he should be assisting Esther with her needs. This time his quality of life would have to be administered too. It would do both of them no good if Ernie was to falter because he felt he had no options available to him. He was coming home to his wife that was slowly dying and was making it as best she could under the circumstances. They would both have to learn to compromise. Esther would have to solely practice in the household chores. This would have to be accomplished without immediately calling Ernie for backup. Ernie would have to learn to stand back and let Esther take control of what she could.

WORKING TOGETHER

Having two head strong individuals wanting to run their lives their way was a recipe for attacks on each other's character. Both of them were being in the needy role. It was also confusing at times for their children to know which one required the attention first. Lines had to be drawn so everyone was clear on duties made and completed. No battles were going to take place, just common courtesy to each.

Ernie would over the course of many years have more important stints put in place. Esther would have many more frightening MRI's and tests to complete. As usual the girls would pitch in and put themselves aside and do what was right for Ernie and Esther. Usually this need to care for them was done without pressure. We would feel satisfied with the outcome. There were occasions of course when the role was taken on because of obligation and necessity. There were times when being and doing right just would happen at the wrong time. The frustration of it all would become annoying. It would feel like to many awful days compared to many cheerful ones. A clear head was clouded with constant worry and sadness. Optimism once became doubtful. This dread was following me and the other girls around every corner. Every move made seemed to be attached to the invisible thread that kept us adhered to this deadly disease Cancer. The weight of this confusion could be very controlling and draining. My mind would play cruel tricks with me in my dreams. I could see a horizon where Esther was going to prosper. This space was full of promise and a bright existence. Then I would wake up to the gloom of not knowing how many more hours or days she would be here in the present world. This chilling place was full of pain and doubt.

Criticism would come from those who knew no better. My children would see my face with more tears than with smiles. I am sorry for that and it saddens me. I want to pass on my happiness for what we have gotten to experience with both Ernie and Esther. When I see and think of them I feel overwhelmed with the sheer triumph they both have endeared. Why do some seem to struggle when others do not?

RHEA'S GRADUATION

The year is 2008 and my daughter is graduating high school. This is when I really observed Esther's failing first hand. Ernie and Esther had been invited to come and celebrate this monumental occasion with us. We were all so excited to have both sets of Grandparents here. To see my daughter get rewarded for her achievements over the past twelve years was heartwarming. I, along with several other women were in charge of the decorating committee for Grad. We all had worked countless hours. The colored sparkles for the tables made each one glow. Delicate lighting circled meticulously on willows painted in white. Tables and chairs all pushed perfectly around the tables with eight or ten place sittings. The entrances were enhanced with large decorations for all to notice the Graduation class enter the field house. Center pieces were strategically placed on all the beautiful tables. This was a very big under taking for the couple of women who worked feverishly on this project. With it finally all complete, we could revel in our work and enjoy the day ahead.

Grad day was a very busy one. I was up extremely early and back to the Centre. I was to double check that everything was running smoothly. My daughter was getting her doo done. The grandparents were dressed in their finest and ready to par take in the ceremony. They just required a cue from me as to when they could make their entrance into the Bonnyville Centralized High

School. Now that everyone was in orderly fashion we could pace ourselves and find suitable seats for the ceremony.

Arriving early would mean I could get Esther to her seat before all others were entering the gymnasium. Also this way I could have Esther to the washroom before any special awards were delivered. With that duty taken care of we began to get comfortable for the program ahead. I excitedly noticed that all the fancy graduates were forming a straight line to enter the gymnasium. Esther whispered to me that she absolutely required the restroom once more. Without being nasty about the situation, we promptly shuffled in front of the entire audience towards the exit. The ladies washroom was out of the Gymnasium and down a stretched hallway. I proceeded to get Esther there with urgency. I was speculating that the Graduates were about to enter the Gym with all its awaiting guests. I nervously and patiently waited for Esther to appear from the washroom. The Graduates were steadily starting to enter where the parents, Grandparents, friends and family were watching with anticipation. Esther quietly came to meet me. I was flustered by the side at the door. I had to whisper and directly tell her that, "We have to wait until the progression of students is complete." Esther needed my assistance back to her seat, which was across the floor and in the front on the opposite side. I did not regrettably get to see my daughter enter the Gym as I was outside with Esther.

I was pissed at the situation and not at her. Once all the Graduates had taken their place on the large stage, I helped Esther get to her assigned seat. I was a little perturbed for the inconvenience that had occurred. It was just very bad timing for washroom duty. Esther and I were in a conundrum that had put us both in bad light. I was angry that her bladder had once again made it to the front of the line and everything else became second. Esther, no doubt was embarrassed because her body decided not to cooperate and had failed her one more time.

I had waited twelve years to see my daughter walk that long trail to the center of her school. I had missed it by pure minutes. My selfishness had made me angry. I did not want to feel this resentment on a very special day. As the long day progressed, Esther and I would make many more calls to the now familiar washroom together. What became clear to me on that particular day was that Esther was requiring more assistance with walking. Her bodily functions were starting to interrupt her scheduled daily routines. I was witnessing situations now where the one in control was definitely not Esther, us or her professionals. The strong disease, known as Cancer was becoming the host of Esther's body.

Esther and Ernie at Bonnyville

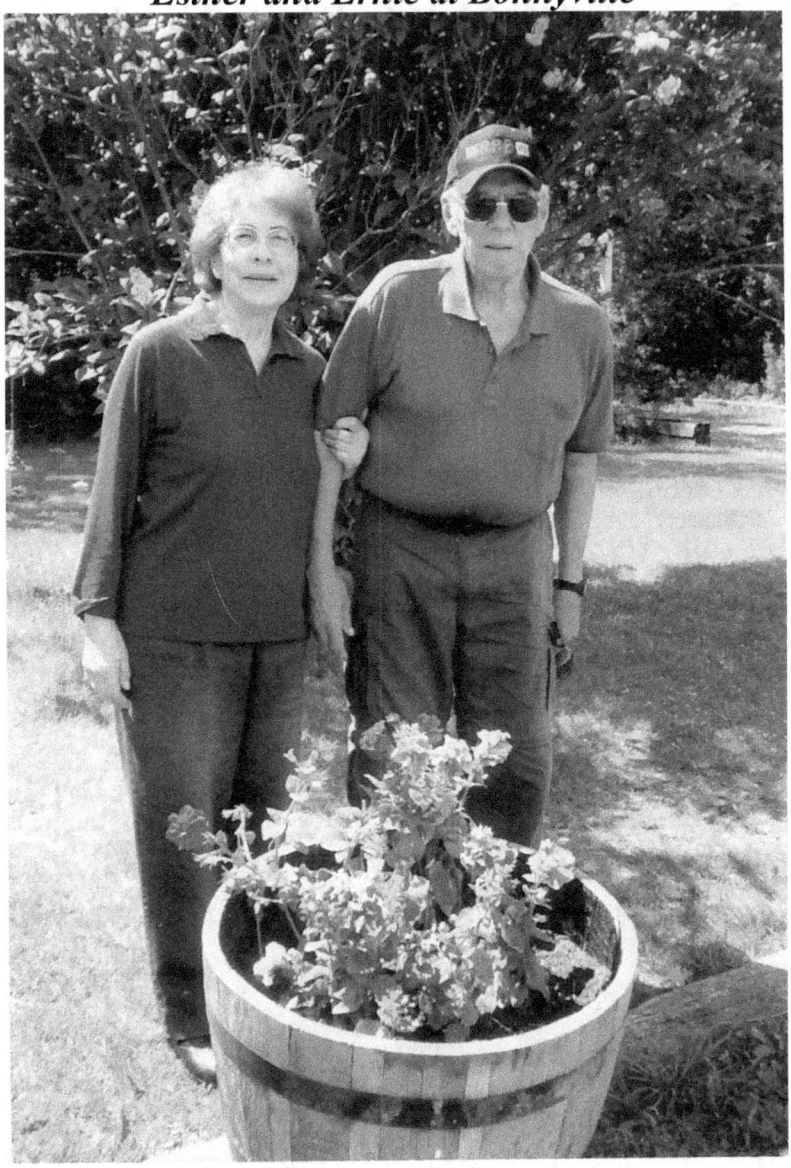

-My jaws are terribly sore and I am very tired today. I am trying to use my mouth guard for a while. I might have to start wearing it at night as I know I am sleeping with my mouth open.

-I am having trouble with noise in my ear. I cannot sleep well.

-I am having a lot of nerve pain and this makes me so mad. Thank goodness I don't show my nerves. I feel like I am shaking on the inside and I am so very cold.

-This house work takes forever but I can't afford to have my house keeper all over again. Then it might not help me out mentally or physically. I have to keep going on.

-Thank goodness Ernie could do the work on the plumbing in this house. I could have never done it. I hope he can outlast me. He is not very well and I am worried about all these renters and the house. I can hardly sleep worrying about it all. I'll have to move if he gets really sick or dies.

What a terrible thought but I will share it with you now.

-February Second, 1999, I was up at six thirty a.m. for my first appointment at eight thirty a.m. The recent results were good and now I have a new eye prescription because of my eye surgery. I have mild Cataracts starting. I had an M.R.I. at eleven a.m. at the Cross Cancer Clinic.

-I believe Cin (daughter's dog) is part human. Some of the things they had her doing; their dog has got feelings like a human being.

-Ernie had stress test today. Thank goodness he did ok. He will go to work on Monday. He is very happy about it. I don't blame him for being so happy. He was really keyed up about it.

-Get the good and bad in this deal. That's life for you. But it is great to have life.

-Up at six forty five a.m., June Twenty Second, 1999, Ernie talked to specialist at four p.m. He said my condition is still the same. I thought it would be worse as I seem so tired and seem to be walking worse.

-I think I am having a slight Heart Attack. I have been having some sharp pains around my heart for the past few weeks. Last night it was sharper in bed after I slept.

-The pain was a little bit in my fingers. I don't want to go to the hospital as it is cold there.

-A friend phoned today to ask about Ernie. She meant well but got me so upset. She talked about all the people who had died and were dying. After the call I started to cry and Ernie was so upset. We went to bed at seven thirty p.m.

-I took two extra pain pills before church, three with Morphine. I usually take six pain pills, two Morphine pills and four Ibuprofen per day.

-Noticed Ernie was facing her at a distance and she was facing him. I am sure they were both looking at one another. If I die they can stretch up a friendship.

-At least she has a good reputation. We have had our talks about this. I told him to be extra careful with women now that he has had a Heart Attack. Some women would love him to get what he has. He says he won't but when you are lonely

it's hard not to be taken advantage of. I think he will be careful.

-Ernie is feeling sick to his stomach. I said it might be the pain pills and he is going to stop taking them for a few days. His back and legs were very painful and was limping some. I am really worried about him.

-He will go and see the specialist tomorrow for his wrist. Hope he will be okay as he goes alone, as I will just be in the way.

-Saw doctor today and he said I should walk two blocks a day. I have told my friends not to mention to others the pain I am in. I don't want others looking at me in a strange way.

-I went for coffee with a dear friend today. We had a good visit and I could not ask for a better friend.

-Home care nurse came and I told her I had a terrible dry mouth and I guess it is due to the medicine. I will get a spray for my mouth.

-My weight was down three pounds. I wasn't

surprised as I didn't feel like eating much. I lost three pounds in one week.

-Came home and took a laxative and such and threw it all up, all of today's food.

-I was so cold; I had to wear leggings under my slacks. We went to my daughters for supper and it was so cold I had to get an extra sweater to wear. I also got a quilt to put on me. It's not even winter and I feel so darn cold. I am sitting here writing with heat packs on my back. This is sure hard to take.

-I am so cold, I feel like I have a million needles poking me all the time. I have to go through this for family and myself.

-I told health nurse today that I could no longer take anti-depressant. It was so terrible with a dry throat. I thought I was going to choke to death. I was so tired on it. I thought I cannot live this way.

-I have not walked all week. My back, hip and leg were so sore. When the health nurse came I just broke down.

-My daughter stopped at noon and gave me heck for letting the pain get ahead of me. I just never took other pills with Ernie coming home and such. My daughter was going to get a hold of the doctor and see if they will put me on a spasm pill. She told me to lie down all afternoon.

-Carmen came by herself today to visit. She says no one really knows how she feels. I agree as no one really knows how I feel. I know she is scared and worried about herself and her family. Life deals us a rough hand sometimes. Thank god she has children and they are as old as they are. I think why God gives me all this sickness. Just leave my children alone.

-My hip and legs are very sore but I wanted to go with my close friend for coffee. I complained to her and only I could with her. I thought I would try to phone my specialist in Edmonton. I am wondering if there is something else wrong.

-Carmen phoned in the evening and we had a good talk. I told her to tell us her problems and not keep them to herself. I might cry but I want to know how she feels. I have told her so much of my

problems.

-I saw a Cancer Specialist today on April Eighteenth, 2000. At two fifteen p.m. I had an M.R.I. I always hate going through this, but I have to.

-I will have an Extensive Bowel exam on May Fourth, 2000. I cannot eat for two and a half days before exam. I will have a terrible time.

-I spilt a glass of milk and then a glass of juice on the table today. I was so fed up with myself.

-I woke up at four thirty this morning and couldn't go back to sleep. I felt I couldn't breathe right and still feel this way.

-I heard on the radio today about a Brownvale resident that died at the age of sixty two with a Brain Tumor. It gave me a terrible feeling. I am thinking I may be that age and dead. I must get my mind busy and not think about it.

-The Home Care Nurse came in the morning to check my urine again. I am up so much in the night.

-I showed the grandchildren how they could

eat Rosehips, Cranberries and Blueberries to survive in the bush. This could be the last time outside in the fall together.

-This cooking is so damn hard on me. Wish I could win the 649 lottery and get a cook.

-There is so much work for Ernie to do here and plus the old garage. I hope he lives to be old and get some new joints repaired and live without pain. He sure works hard for all this life.

-I saw a couple we know as of late and she wanted to know why I use a cane. I just said I had not been feeling well. Lately I use this answer on a lot of people now. It seems to shut them up.

-I went to the dentist yesterday and it was another big bill. My teeth have been falling apart since the radiation.

-I had a lot of pain in my head today and took four extra pain pills. I went for coffee and tried not to think about all the tests on Tuesday at the Cancer Clinic.

-I cannot seem to write very often anymore. I

woke up at 6:00 a.m. and thought at first it was eight and then couldn't go back to sleep. I woke up at two thirty, four thirty and six a.m. and then at seven fifteen a.m. I hope my kidneys are ok. I asked the first Cancer Specialist what should happen to me and she said that the kidneys go first.

-I have to stay strong through it. It is hard on my family to see me this way.

-Working on the quilt seems like such a big job. My hand is so sore and eyes blurry.

-I get so lonely for a visit with my children, even if the visit is short.

-The eye Doctor says my right eye is worse than the last time I saw him on November Twenty Eighth, 2001. It is the start of Cataracts. The eye sight may change again soon. I don't know what to do.

-We had assessments about our backs today. Not good news. He stated that there was a fifty-fifty chance of having a good back operation. He thought we should just leave things the way they are. We are in such pain.

-An old friend joined me for coffee today. I was taken back as she was asking me some very personal questions about my health. She should be more careful not to hurt people's feelings.

-My two sisters came to the house to wish me a Happy Birthday. When they left early I became upset. We hardly had a chance to visit. I was so looking forward to seeing them. I broke down and cried.

-I was so constipated, having a terrible time with this. This all makes me so mad.

-It is very quiet here by myself. Sometimes I feel very alone.

-My sister and I went out for supper. We had a nice talk about our families. We talked about our mother and how our home life was growing up. We admire my mother so much now as we are older and understand what she was going through.

-My friend called me for coffee but my teeth were in so much pain. I just didn't think I could go. This is the first time I turned down a chance to

go out.

-My jaw and teeth bother me every day. I keep going but so hard to. My mouth was sore which makes me mad as it's hard to deal with the pain and all the rest. I try to keep my mind off of it.

-My freezing in my teeth came out about three p.m. The pain was terrible, just about went out of my mind. I am up every night at three thirty a.m. and have to take two more pain pills to go back to sleep.

-My good friend did not want to have coffee with me today as she has a cold and is very worried and concerned not to pass anything on to me.

-In 1941, I was one year old and the bombing of Pearl Harbor happened. Today I hear about the World Trade Centre and such. I just felt like I wanted to be around family in such sad times. Family is the most important now.

-Saw a Specialist about my jaw and teeth problems. He thought it was mostly my jaw causing the pain. He prescribed a prescription and took it for two days and became terribly sick

to my stomach. I am not going through this again where I was sick for ten months straight coming home from the hospital.

-I ate Christmas dinner without being sick, since my doctor changed my medicine.

-I went to bed early and watched some T.V. to bring in the New Year 2002. These old ladies live a more exciting life than me. I don't want to become a widow and find out.

-It is so hard for me to see Uncle John at the Sutherland Nursing Home. I keep seeing myself like this.

-I have to stop thinking so negative. I need to think positive. I wish I could be more so. I worry more than the average person as I probably have too much time to think.

-My worst day of the week is Saturday. I always feel lonely and without direction.

-Wednesday night I was too tired to get in and out of the tub. I could hardly walk. Wish I felt better about camping. It has been so cold and

windy that I am not looking forward to it. The motels can be very cold too but at least you can have a decent bath and curl your hair easier. I don't like it. It's my last trip this way. Both ways are very tiring but I would like to get away from here for a while.

-Ernie had a talk with my neighbor bringing me such bad news. She told me of seven people that had either died or are dying of Brain Cancer. She goes into such detail. She said she was sorry.

-It was a bad day on Tuesday. Almost every magazine I read had a Cancer story in it.

-Had a backache all the way home and trouble breathing. Eight hours in the truck was enough.

-Ernie is not feeling well today. He says he is shaky and weak. He has said this several times in the past months. Hope he is ok.

-Had a big supper and threw it all up. What a mess, all over the toilet and floor.

-Ernie brought over Cinnamon (daughters dog). Said she wanted to come over and see Grandma. Ernie loves all these animals.

-I keep waking up so early at five thirty a.m. I am up once a night and don't go to sleep until twelve a.m. and I am so tired by five p.m. I can hardly keep going. I have tried to cut down on OxyContin by two pills. I get up at six thirty a.m. so as not to think about what could happen to me.

-Ernie went to see the Doctor today. He fell down the steps to the office. It's a wonder he didn't break a knee. Ernie got the paper and it said our hospital was changing over February Fourteenth, 2003. It has made all of us very sad.

-Ernie is in so much pain today. He is working on his truck out in the open. I sure wish I had a garage for him to work in. When I win a million I will get him one.

-Ernie called Carmen to tell her he just couldn't make it to her place for Christmas. He wanted to so badly but was in just too much pain and misery. It has been just an on and off trip. Now it is off.

-I can't seem to get another diary like this to write in. So I don't know what I will do.

-Made pickled eggs today, these are like what my dad used to make when I was small.

-Ernie drove himself to the Grimshaw Hospital. He packed his toothbrush and stuff from home as he must have known he was not returning. The Doctor admitted him. Ernie was in rough shape. He could hardly breathe and was in terrible pain and his shoulder was so sore.

-We went to see Ernie at the hospital at eleven a.m. He was much better and could eat a little today. At seven p.m., Ernie had made a remarkable difference in his health in just one day. Ernie was a lot more cheerful. Doctor took him off the drip and just gave him a shot in the arm.

-My son in law was going to relieve a family friend at work up in Fort Nelson. Then this person could come home and be with his ailing mother who is my close friend and wait for her to die. It is so hard on everyone.

ENDING ESTHER'S MEMORY

JOURNAL

ESTHER AND ERNIE IN FRONT OF HAAS AUTO

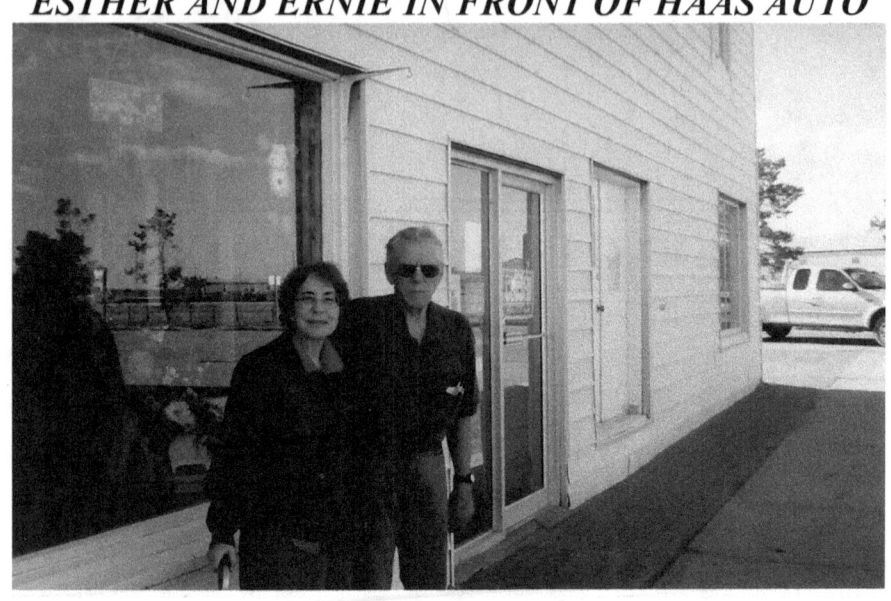

ERNIE AND ESTHER IN GRIMSHAW

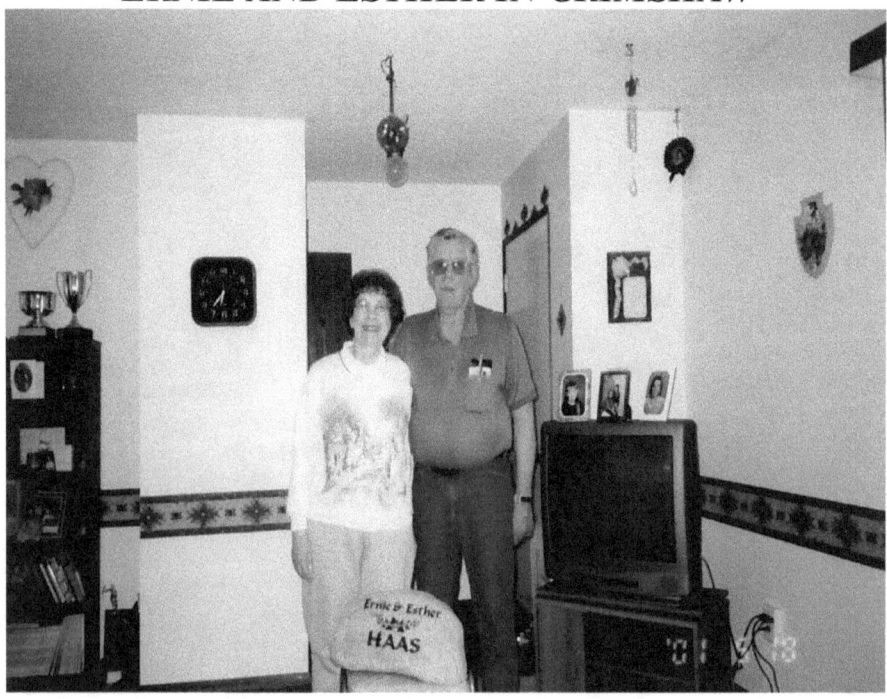

ESTHER'S BODY SLOWING DOWN

Esther was increasingly having much difficulty going up the red carpeted stair case to her bedroom and bathroom. The carpet on the entire upper level made it extremely hard for Esther to grasp her footing. Her right leg was dragging some; she would catch herself tripping from her foot connecting with the unforgiving carpet. It seemed at times that she walked as if she had had a stroke on that side of her body. The Brain was damaged on the left side of her head, which affected the right side of her body. A strange and peculiar thing when your body reacts to trauma on the opposite side of the body. Her jaw was becoming a source of agony. The gag reflex was not letting her eat and swallow properly. Her chocking was becoming more of a threat. Her eyesight was ever changing. Her hearing became more impaired. Her right hand was gradually getting weaker. The grasp was delayed when going to hold something. The hips were constantly with aches and pains. The Bladder was becoming more insufficient. Her body was just plainly not listening to the signals put forth. Her requests were vacant without any response. Esther's mind was complete with accuracy. Her body however was showing clear signs of shut down.

It was becoming more and more prevalent for Ernie and the girls to watch Esther more closely. The strain to give her baths, even with the aid of a bath lift was becoming too much. Esther would get a portable potty put in the living room. She could at least relieve herself when Ernie was not around to help her up the stairs. Her bladder also needed to flush more often and quickly. With the potty close by she didn't have the worry of not making it on time. Once she was awake in the morning and dressed she would continue to stay on that same level until later in the day when Ernie would arrive home.

Many times Esther would find herself in situations where she would become helpless and at the mercy of others. She was in her garden admiring the vegetables when without warning she just simply fell to the dirty ground. She could not find the strength or energy to manipulate herself up from the soil. She tried every possible way she could think of to distance herself from the dirt. With every try she became more and more exhausted. She was withered now with fright and panic. With no phone handy, she was fixated to this patch of earth until Ernie arrived home many hours later.

The entire family was in Ernie and Esther's oversized large backyard having a game of ball. Esther in her youth played Fast Ball on many winning teams. She was very talented in this sport. It got the best of her just being a spectator. She wanted to be a participant and show us just how well she could still manage a glove and bat. She got all lined up with the long hard wooden bat and the white leather ball was thrown. She swung the forceful bat and made a direct contact and connected with the round ball.

The ball went flashing through the air. Esther then lost her balance and immediately fell to the grassy lawn. We all rushed to her side with concern in our worried eyes. As we stared down upon her, she smiled and said, "I have fallen and I can't get up." Our stern faces had been charged with laughter. We knew she was fine. We all found room in our aching hearts to know that laughter was a main ingredient to staying strong and solid. To cry and laugh is human. We would have our share of both.

Ernie was requested to go see his Medical Doctor in Grimshaw. He had a multitude of blood tests completed. He was given the news a short while later that his blood count was extremely low. He would be required to ingest iron pills for a month to build the blood count back to normal. Esther is truly concerned and realizes that Ernie is slightly worried about these findings. Ernie's father had similar blood related problems. Leukemia was the blood disorder that his father was ailing from. Ernie would comply with his Doctor's wishes. Ernie and Esther were on a multitude of different medications. They would try their hardest to keep each other informed. When one or the other had a doctor's appointment scheduled they would go as a pair. Two sets of ears would hopefully grasp what the other individual may not. They would touch base every day as to their health concerns in case of an emergency. Even having one of their daughters present at these informative meetings would help with the instructions given from the Professionals. Just another person's perception could clear up any confusion that perhaps was unclear.

WORDS OF FRUSTRATION

The girls would periodically join Ernie and Esther at their home over noon hour breaks. Discussions of doom and gloom at this time of day could be disheartening for their daughters. They would have to continue back to their jobs and put on smiles when their hearts were full of sadness. Hearing how poorly they felt would absolutely cause stress for the rest of the day. There were plenty of moments when Ernie and Esther were not joining forces in their partnership. The harshness of their accusations could set each other off into insulting each other's pride. Downright nasty and vicious was being served as the main course for today. Snakes venom was being spit in every direction. If you were the unlucky one to enter their domain today, you had to be ready to put on your armor and enter the battle field. These were the frustrating times that were sure to surface. The boldness of words were stated but were said with regret. Each was condemned to falter. The heat of these interferences would linger in the air. They were using each other's forms as punching bags. It was hard to witness these heated discussions. It surely was not right to commit such damaging insults. We hurt and use the ones that are closest to us. You disrupt the ones you love the most. Oddly enough these are the very individuals that will forgive you of all your wickedness. We all need to vent at certain times. The damaging words they used seemed to apply to their better understanding of one another. What ever worked for them was not for me to judge. I was not the one walking in their footsteps. It would seem that their love however unkindly at points just made them more united.

Esther's younger brother became a main topic of conversation one day. His name wasn't brought up much. He was however mentioned at one of these lunches. Esther's eyes formed tears, as she had mostly wished she could have helped him out more. She didn't have much to offer him in the way of shelter. When she finally did possess her own dwelling, the infrastructure was so very small. She gathered at his older age that boredom would overtake him. He was used to his life of freedom. Esther would tell her daughter that at times she felt tangled between her two families of siblings. She would place roots when she could. Then there was the extended family that she would see less often. With eleven brothers and sisters, you could picture how one sibling could be squeezed in or out depending on the situation. You might not be noticed at all. Esther felt so indebted to her sisters. Her mother was crippled and could not raise her and her younger brother and sister. Esther was so grateful for one sister in particular. She was older than Esther and took care of her when needed. Esther would struggle with the thought of never being able to pay her back for her generosity. Esther's wellbeing was never brought to the surface. She didn't want them to feel as they had not done their best. Esther knew of course that her entire family did what they could for her at the time.

BLOOD TRANSFUSIONS

Christmas of 2001 would become a true pleasure for the family, as Esther and Ernie had survived another year. It was a huge surprise for all when my family showed up unexpectedly at their front door. Ernie had heard various rumors that we might be making an appearance. He never uttered a word to anyone. This exciting moment had given Ernie a little boost to feel better as he was under the weather physically. He was extremely weak, pale and very tired. The color of his skin was taking on a grayish tone. He was sent to the hospital immediately for some blood tests and foot x-ray. His blood count was extremely low. Six was his count, when the normal is about fourteen. He also was informed at the hospital that he had a severely broken toe. He had been lifting an old heavy exercise bike up a flight of stairs when he suddenly dropped this awkward machine on his foot. Due to his low energy he was required to become a patient at the hospital for two days. He would be induced with two blood transfusions. This course of action was hopefully going to bring his mobility to better heights. The doctors seemed to reason that Ernie must be bleeding on the inside. Ernie would always try to find humor in a negative situation. He decided that he must have a leak somewhere on his fractured body and just not sure where it was going. Four more units of rich blood would be replenished into his slow moving body. This would definitely explain why he was just not himself. His productivity was being measured. His lazy body would know show signs of increased strength.

TIME TICKING AWAY

Esther had been managing on her own at home with help from her daughters, husband, friends and health care workers. Esther had functioned for nine years relatively fair. She had surpassed her diagnosis of death. Her two to five years of survival was marveled. By all rights, she was to be dead four years ago. To have her here with us at this point in our lives was a true miracle. Esther had got to celebrate more births within the family and sadly witness the deaths of her close friends. Some of these people were not even ill when she was diagnosed with Cancer. They had lost to death quickly. This was always very hard on Esther and Ernie. Her own mortality always came into play when funerals came and went. Esther would not attend any of these good byes, as she just couldn't bare the sadness everyone felt, especially her own. The guilt of surviving loved ones sentenced to death like her was very daunting.

Esther and Ernie planted their special flowers every summer in the beds waiting with fresh black dirt. The Petunias were always bright with color and placed in the designed flower beds. The deck would supply hundreds of these hardy blossoms. The covered deck would let in just the right amount of sun for heat but suffice as shelter from the bright rays. Esther especially would absorb the warmth from the sun on her pale soft skin. Esther's yard had become her haven, her Eden on earth. The giant yard gave her a chance to connect with her world on a physical and mental level. Everything she saw or heard became fragments of a picture she would not want to let go of. The small birds singing, the wind slowly blowing in her face, the fragrance off the new buds and the feeling of her heart beating would be lost soon enough. She would not let these precious moments slip past. To her the yard was just a blessing and gave her mind a place to drift and surround herself with peace. Her moments on the deck were splendid and treasured as she never knew when the gift would end. Esther would get to enjoy her wonderful back yard for another day.

The family would treasure one more Christmas and celebrate the New Year with thanks. Every holiday was to be locked away in our memories. When Esther was around, her presence was always felt. She was not meek and mild; she was vibrant and had electricity you could feel. She could make a room come to an abrupt stop with her orders. Or she brought passion and complexity to her tasks that she would take on gingerly. She wore bright colors, which added to her vibrant personality. Esther took extra time every day to brighten her face with her favorite makeup. She knew it was a hassle and didn't have to but took pride in her appearance. She would enter her bathroom with a cup of steaming tea or coffee and start the process. Even in her darkest hours she still tried to brighten the picture.

Esther was in her tenth year now, still fighting the beast, known as Cancer. Her cold body was always covered with layers of clothing. She wore long johns, extra under shirts and cozy slippers just to try to stay warm. The heating pad and heater bags for the microwave had become her source of internal heat.

THE DEMON CANCER

Ernie was being pressured to become the complete care giver. The needful health nurses were up until this point giving Esther her baths once a week in the upstairs bathroom. Esther looked so forward to this cleansing that they provided. The nurses were providing Esther the opportunity to still keep her dignity in tack. With them supplying the routine of bathing, Ernie or the girls did not have to see Esther's tired body parts withering away. Her muscles and skin were becoming limp without having mobility to exercise. Her small droopy breasts were not requiring the bra once needed. The nurses were accommodating Esther her last bit of privacy. Esther tried to shield this one task from the family as much as possible. Everyone involved in Esther's care had to face the fact that the process of bathing Esther in her own environment was becoming too difficult and unsafe for them to continue. Esther's daughters would start to assist her and complete her personal needs. During the day one of the girls were able to continue with her care. At night however Ernie became the sole provider. He was capable of making three meals a day. He would assist Esther to the portable toilet when needed. He was discarding of waste and cleaning messy portable toilets. Ernie was helping Esther with her ensemble for the day. He would assist with the undoing of her garments at night. At the end of a very long shift he would still manage with her day end rituals and cleaning schedule. Ernie's nights were interrupted with giving support to Esther's bodily functions. The days spent completing the same endless chores became a job of unwanted necessity. Ernie complied because of duty and love. Esther accepted because of no choice and love.

All this gathered tension, stress and tiredness was building up like a volcano getting ready to burst. Esther would become a snake just waiting to strike. She would get angry with Ernie for the slightest mishap. The doors on the cupboard were not closed properly. The butter wasn't placed on the table for supper. Ernie would just sit down ready to relax and enjoy a meal when Esther would need a glass of tepid water. The water could not be too cold because of her tender teeth. Every little thing was made into something bothersome. Her tone of voice would become so aggressive and vocally loud. Ernie just seemed to irritate Esther constantly. The sights of him in her company just become her focal point to belittle him. Esther's outbursts were volatile and hugely exaggerated. Ernie would comply with all of Esther's demands as he was trying the best he could to do right by her. He would at times just not be able to control his frustration. Ernie would get so hurt that he would have to physically leave the premises for a period. Ernie would lose his patience and undoubtedly would say and do things that were not appropriate. There were days when they were stripped of their defenses. They both had endeared enough and didn't have the muscle to face another day. When Ernie and Esther would revolt in front of us, it was painful to watch. To see your parents attacking each other mentally becomes disheartening. Their behavior was unacceptable. Our parents would have never wanted their daughters to live with this kind of cruelty from their mate. This storm that affected their personalities and bombarded their space was tolerated only because of their union. Yet I could always see the love shining through the cracks constantly. The progression from toleration to torment I might not understand. I was witness to their signs of commitment, gratitude and true love. This is how they chose to survive the wickedness of Cancer. It worked for them.

The extreme days with built up anxiety for Esther became more frequent with time. She was becoming aware that continuing to live at home was becoming a burden on the family. The daughters were supplying aid when it was possible for them. They also had jobs and families to tend too. Ernie's health and well fare was also a concern at this point. He was becoming extremely exhausted and spent. Ernie was losing his spunk and humor. His sparkle was dimming. His smile was nowhere in sight. His days like Esther's were full of similarity and repetitiveness. Their lives had become full of the sameness every day.

Ernie would surely take all of Esther's grumpiness, if it meant one more single day she could spend with the family. He could go on and on with these fretful days if that is what it would take to crush the Cancer. I would tell him often that Esther would get rough and heated with him because he is the closest person she had. She knows you will forgive her indiscretions. They would fight some good fights but when it was all said and done their bond for each other is what kept her going and fighting. Ernie would never give up on his Esther even when she was downright frigid. I would catch myself being jealous of their continued support. Hopefully I had a man in my life that would not break when he needed to bend. Would my own family give so unselfishly if I was in the same position? Would my own sisters stand by me and not let me fight alone. Ernie and Esther had a true connection even through the panic and desperation they felt.

A PLACE TO LIVE

Esther and Ernie were starting to seriously examine their options for different living arrangements. The Heritage Towers in Peace River was a twenty minute drive from Grimshaw. This place could home both of them, if required to do so. The huge building was adjacent to the wondering hills which gave you a beautiful view. Many names registered familiar to Esther and Ernie, they were advertised on the doors that were closed down the existing hallway. They offered so many things that Esther would find inviting. Esther being the social butterfly would have her days filled with numerous activities. There was however just one deterrent; Esther could not sufficiently remove herself from the premises without support. Should the building be on fire, a natural or manmade disaster take place and she had no one to aid her, she would essentially go down with the ship. The Towers was not able to fulfill her needs. Of course this all made sense and we were on to the next possible opening.

To buy a condo in Grimshaw was probably a fine idea. They would have to sell their existing dwelling first and how long would that process take? What should happen if Ernie passed away and Esther was left in the condo alone? Would the money they made from the sale of the house be sufficient to purchase the condo and keep Esther afloat financially? Would she be able to sustain living in the condo under her own accord? There just were so many scenarios to think of. Your head could start spinning with the variations of circumstances that could happen. The right choice could just seem bad when you took into account all that could go possibly wrong.

The Berwyn Lodge was an acceptable place to look into. Esther new many of the residents that occupied the comfortable rooms there. She had heard that many seemed to thrive here. The meals offered seemed to be better than most. The small town of Berwyn was only ten minutes away. There were rooms available immediately and the Lodge was close to home. Or they could just stay put in their existing house. They could continue to function with things the way they stood.

Over the next several months Esther would contemplate what she should do. They would bounce back and forth from one decision to another. One day they were definitely moving and the next was the complete opposite. Ernie and Esther would get the girls to arrange viewings and meetings to see houses, condos and Lodges. There seemed to be no perfect solution to their dilemma. All Esther new for certain was her body was starting to falter more with each passing day. She had to make a big decision and soon.

However none of these assisted living arrangements were including Ernie. He would not be swayed to pursue any new address to fit anyone's desires. He was absolutely, positively, not being urged to move anywhere. This discussion was closed. If any moves were made to accommodate Esther, she would be arriving somewhere alone. He would pack, load and sign on the dotted line when necessary but he was most certainly going to be a visitor and not an attendee. He could pretend, show interest and even view these locations of living but we all new very well indeed that he would not leave his quarters until he was literally pushed out the door.

THE BERWYN LODGE

Esther's decision to advance quickly into the Berwyn Lodge was driven by urgency. She could feel the pressure from all sides. Her inner and outer circle were vocalizing "this is the right decision for you and your family".

Esther had massive courage to vacate her home. She felt protected there against intruders of the mortal kind. See took that first shuffled gait and did not look back for fear of losing her nerve. She put the troublesome presence away and brought out her reserve of strength. This gallant decision would be hers alone.

This peculiar life she was invested in was not at all perfect. It could still remain her property at this point. She would be making the important calls for herself. The choice to make ground breaking decisions may seep away with time. She would muster up what she still had and arrange the details when and while she still could. She was moving without Ernie by her side. This was the right prescription for everyone involved. Her conscience was ordering her to do this deed. Her heart however felt much sorrow and defeat. She would be leaving so much of her existence behind.

Esther had a somewhat impaired judgment about the Berwyn Lodge. She heard from some of her close advisers that this is what she needed to accomplish. Esther was guided to believe that she would be making this fundamental sacrifice for her family. She was tackled and bombarded with this decision when she was at her most vulnerable. Esther was entering a facility that was going to in reality bring her spirit way down and could ultimately defeat her. The Lodge itself was ran appropriately. They conducted themselves with all the diligence expected of a long term facility. It was functioning and equipped with all that it should. Esther was however the youngest person living in the Lodge by far. Some of the elders were in better shape physically than Esther. Her days were filled with confusion and regret and were extremely long and boring. She longed terribly for the scenery of her busy yard. Visitors were a welcome site and a distraction from the normality that was present. With much luck she would be venturing home on weekends to inhale the senses while she could.

Ernie was catching up on his much needed sleep but found the house exceptionally quiet. His routine was in disarray and he found it hard to step outside from his diligent schedule.

Esther was barely surviving at the Lodge due to the constant handicaps she saw in others around her. This sea of unwell and diseased patients around her made Esther feel doomed. She was feeling staggered and useless. The burden of Cancer was all too real here. There was so much time to contemplate the future because of the simple structure. The limits of life all around her was enough a reason to give up on this battle all together.

Esther was entering her third month at the Lodge. A local male doctor that was accustomed to seeing Esther on a regular basis stopped by for a casual visit. He with great puzzlement, said flatly to Esther, "what are you doing, you don't belong here." That was all Esther needed to hear to be vindicated. Ernie and one of the twins along with her daughter rushed to Esther's aid. They packed up her solemn room with quick aggressiveness. Esther returned to her splendid home with green grass and flowers with bright pastel petals. Her house was so welcoming with soothing sounds and intoxicating smells that she had missed so much. She loved this home so dearly.

BACK AT EDEN

Being back at her salvation meant certain changes
were in store. Having the closest washroom on the upper
level would just not suffice anymore. The portable toilet
would certainly continue to be placed in the handy living
room for the entirety of Esther's stay. For Esther to have
complete privacy, a long shower curtain was placed
between the solid hallway walls. If she were busy with
private matters she could simply pull the curtain closed.
The walker would be her source of mobility on this floor.
She could place her water, phone and heater bags in the
basket attached to the walker. The wheel chair became a
valuable tool and was an irreplaceable machine. To push
Esther for long distances, the wheel chair just made so
much more sense. It put less strain on everyone including
Esther. The walker would be tugged at times as it just
didn't have the mobility and ease that the wheelchair
could provide. It would take time and effort to adjust to
new procedures. Some extreme anxiety would occur
during this radical phase. Ernie would continue to do the
chores as needed. Esther's bed was immediately placed
in the center of the spacious living room on the main
level. A satisfactory square night stand was placed by the
bed. An adequate toilet was also aligned with in arms
reach. Her TV was centered at the far end of the room for
clear viewing. Several chairs would surround the
perimeter of the large room. Her clothes were arranged in
a nearby hall closet. Esther would now have the

conformability of her necessities close at hand. If any visiting was to be had it was assigned to the kitchen. The living room was off limits to everyone except her family.

Ernie's portable bed, known as the couch was to become accustomed to their original bedroom. Esther would now solely occupy the main floor. She would rarely see the upper level. If the need arose for her to move up stairs the assistance of the health belt was to come into play. This was to be placed around Esther's waist for support and security. The lower level was basically not obtainable. She was still able to glance and scan her surroundings through the clear patio doors. If the weather was agreeable she could readily enjoy the fresh air by resting outdoors.

On early Sunday mornings Ernie and Esther's son in law and their granddaughter would come and execute a game of cards. They both would relish in these mind games. This strategizing would get rid of the monotony they would both surrender to. This was something pleasant to look forward to. They would enjoy this special time with their youngest granddaughter. It truly was a delight for them.

Ernie would become more secluded from his social life. He now was on a tight schedule. Esther would consume her fruits and fiber along with rich smelling coffee in the mornings. She would reluctantly swallow all her wonderful drugs for pain, anxiety, constipation and swallowing. Her small mouth was like a dry sponge. She would suck on hard candies just to get moisture into her throat. Esther would gradually make her way to the portable potty in her make shift bathroom. Ernie would patiently wait for Esther to vacate her bladder. This process of her completing a bowel movement could literally take from minutes to hours. Air freshener was sprayed to mask unpleasant odors; it lingered around the premises for days. Ernie would without complaining take the pungent waste up stairs to the washroom toilet and discard it. He would replace the mobile toilet seat and be ready for the next facts of life to happen. Role reversal had taken place. He now was the acting mother, nurse, chef, scheduler, delivery person and man of the household. Ernie would gather Esther's clothes for the day and display them like a neat uniform ready for duty. Her daily routine of applying her makeup was tedious and timely. When Ernie new Esther was all in order only then would he leave her at home so he could forge for coffee at the local Mile Zero Inn.

He required these extended breaks during the day to keep his sanity. The customary discussions of normalcy he administered with comfort. Men don't really go into depths about their sorrow. Ernie always gathered his close friends were simply a call away if he required considerate words or actions. Many of his friends had already gone through this passage. The words weren't spoken but care showed on their faces. They would keep a vigil on Ernie.

The evenings were dealt with quickly as Ernie would fall into a deep slumber early. Esther's night process would begin with forcing down all her medicine again. Once her evening ritual was complete then Esther would reluctantly go to her awaiting bed and inspect what was on TV or read to bring on the fatigue. She would patiently wait until eleven p.m. to swallow her needed sleeping pill. Hopefully this little blue powder of sleepiness would prompt hours of rest that she yearned for.

Often through the night Ernie would fall into such a trance of rest that he would miss Esther's calls of need. The practice of taking a little bell to bed became her source of arising Ernie. The jingle would awaken him with a startle. This gentle soft but alarming sound would be enough to alert Ernie. Most nights they were disturbed by Esther's uncooperative bladder. Periodically the damp sheets would have to be exchanged for dry ones. Esther's desire to empty her contained bladder would leak before she could connect with her close potty. Esther would now initiate the use of wearing depends to bed to feel more secure through the night. Hopefully this new addition would comply and add to the demand of sleep they so desperately were searching for.

Esther new that arriving home from the Berwyn
Lodge had put pressure and strain on all her care givers.
Not everyone was as excited about her returning home as
she was. There were the odd few that were disrupted by
her sudden change of heart. Some were not sure she had
made the right choice. Esther was confident that vacating
the Lodge was a small step in the right direction. She
would grant herself permission to grasp at the chance for
whatever peace she could find. It was critical and crucial
for her to be among her family and friends at this time.
Esther new that the past could not be changed and all
interested parties would just have to deal with her
decisions. What she was more interested in was trying to
live the rest of her life to the best of her abilities. Esther
would be facing the beast on her terms from now on. It
wasn't death that she feared most. It was what would take
place before the final moments that concerned her. She
just wanted a chance to tackle a few more card games.
Witness more seasons change. Eat more appetizing foods
and see her family and friends whenever possible. That
wasn't too much to ask, was it? She deserved that much,
damn it.

Esther had the power of her army behind her. We
provided and prolonged her stay at home for one whole
gratifying year. Her determination was satisfied. She had
fought hard for this right. However her time was running
out. It was becoming very apparent that Esther could
cause potential danger to herself and others. Her right

foot and leg were more sluggish. Her right hand was seeing the signs of paralyses. Her sight and hearing was becoming a reminder of the Brain Tumor still imprisoned in her head.

The doctors had issued a current MRI due to the symptoms she was experiencing. The news was a reality that we had lived with daily for eleven years. The stretch of period without her demise had always plagued us but we had gladly accepted the blessing. The MRI was not lying and issued us a warning. The Tumor was alive once more. It was growing again at a fast pace within her delicate Brain.

HEATH CARE

Suitable living arrangements for Esther no longer fitted her needs at home. The family scheduled a meeting and viewing with the heads of Health Care to visit Ernie and Esther. We sequestered the system to see firsthand and up close that Ernie could not physically handle the daily routine with Esther any longer. This particular time the twin daughters were in attendance. We told Ernie with regret that we would not be assisting him in any way while the session was in progress. We absolutely needed the health care people to witness the exertion this had on both Ernie and Esther. The harshness of this left a panic in my body. They would explore how Ernie struggled with the menacing wheelchair. It took all his masculine strength to force the chair into a secured a safe position while in transit. Physically assisting Esther from the confines of the truck seat to placing her in the sturdy wheelchair was so demanding of them both. The perspiration was evident. The pulling, bending and swaying made for sore body parts. All this purposeful strain was not gentle on Ernie's heart. With entry into the house came the removal of Esther's outside clothes. She was then glided into the smaller walker. Esther would show them her procedure for gravitating to the potty. With Ernie's contact it went swifter. On her own, Esther was simply not advancing. The energy they poured out had left them looking pale and weathered.

The Heath Care Professionals could see the grief and

despair in both their eyes. They were admitting whole heartedly to all that we alone cannot make it work anymore. It would be like forcing your foot into the wrong size of shoe. No matter the energy or change in strategy the outcome was the same. The fit was just not right and it hurt. They knew Esther would feel the terror about giving up her home once again. Ernie would have the obsession to always take care of her. With gentle seriousness the experts were completely convinced that Esther was a suitable candidate for Long Term Care. The only problem with that scenario was there were no vacancies available in Grimshaw or Peace River.

These two close towns in the area were considered home. To be placed at any other small town would be like signing a death warrant. The distance would be far and would cause an issue. Contact with family and friends was imperative. The terrible certainty of that happening was a very possible reality. Until a room became suitable and available for Esther she would remain at home. Esther was convinced this was the avenue to pursue. They would wait like so many others trying to get into the care system. Real life had surfaced and shown its many colors today. All the feelings we had held and repressed for so long burst out of us in anger, tears and trembles from sheer frustration. We all feared the end. Was it coming closer? God was whispering her name.

SPRAINED ANKLE

Esther would continue to fill her days and nights at her Eden. Every minute and hour would be a challenge. The girls and Ernie would take it upon themselves to make Esther's world functional. On one of the rare occasions, Esther was up stairs alone. She was shuffling her way to the restroom. Her lazy right foot was dragging and caught her unaware. Esther tumbled to the carpeted floor. Her ankle on the right leg became twisted in the fall and caused her major concern. Her distress was justified. Esther's ankle was badly bruised and sprained. The swollen puffiness was evident. Esther was now at the mercy of others once more. She had become totally dependent on her small reliable army. She would be bound to the wheel chair for a long stretch. Her small bit of independence was stripped. Three weeks of confinement had made her weary and blue. Esther would pour out her frustration and confusion verbally once again. Ernie for the most part would take on all of her waste. He noted Esther without objection. She poured her hot ridden doubt into his hands. She was his gentle and gracious wife when she was wearing her true face. The Tumor was the criminal here. The Cancer in her Brain was affecting many emotional areas. It was hard to distinguish Esther from the expert master working against her Brain from the inside. Interference was made by Ernie before too much damage could occur. He would inflict compassion. We would remind Esther that she was not inferior. Her trepidation did matter. A peaceful escape from daily trials did not always come easily. We would push our strength onto her. The unity of her army prolonged her future.

NEW VISION

The entirety of this lengthy sentence of Esther's cancer was taking a toll on her eyesight. She was having much difficulty adjusting to her ever changing prescription. Esther scheduled an appointment to visit her regular eye doctor. She wanted his expert opinion to see her up close and personal. When she left his professional office, she was very distraught due to the diagnosis that was given to her. The doctor blurted out that she was showing signs of producing Immaculate Degeneration. Basically she was going blind. She should surrender to this outcome and make peace with it. This seemed to be his attitude. He was very blasé about the whole conversation that had taken place. It was beneficial that she seek out another's opinion. This doctor without any previous information immediately issued a statement that contained promise. There was no degeneration that he could gather. The cause for alarm was extreme cataracts progressing on both eyes. Surgery could be done to correct this issue. Esther was relieved. She was disheartened with the lack of manners her first doctor had shown. His Professionalism was truly lacking. He never brought any of his kindness or courtesy to the forefront that day. He had placed her in the ground because of her Cancer. She felt invisible and very small in this big world. On top of everything else she didn't want to cope without her sight. To have her sight gone would be too dramatic to deal with. Esther went on to have her cataracts removed successfully. For the first time in my life and in hers we inhaled the sight of her pretty facial features without large framed glasses. Esther was sixty nine when she became glass less. This oddness kept me glancing at her often. This was such a blessing in her life right now. She could look solely for the first time at objects through her new eyes. The curse though was that the Cancer was brewing again. Esther would have this joy to bask in for only a short while.

ESTHER CHOCKING

Esther and Ernie were having a calm relaxing day. Esther was in her bathroom on the upper floor. They both had noticed earlier though that Esther's breathing was becoming labored. It sounded like fluid was mounting in her lungs. Her strenuous breaths she inhaled made a gurgling pitch. Ernie summoned my twin to leave her place of employment to retreat to their house immediately. Ernie's daughter was tied up with customers and was not convinced that Esther's irregular breathing was an emergency. My twin ordered her eldest daughter to rush to her grandparent's side. Upon entering the house and making her way to the upper level she encountered Esther in full blown out chocking. Esther was gasping and fighting for air to enter her clogged lungs. The thick sticky saliva in her throat had become massive gobs. Esther could not force the extreme fluid out. She was not getting any purposeful air through her panicked lungs. My niece was in command of Esther. Ernie was demanding 911 to formulate an entrance and enforce their life savings sanctions on Esther. Ernie along with my niece were stricken with terrible bouts of worry. The thick fluid was now protruding out of her stretched mouth and nose as the substance had nowhere else to exit without her guidance. Esther's blockage was obstructing the air she beckoned for. This instant required appropriate action now. The ambulance arrived and assessed the situation momentarily. My niece was bold and in all her forwardness said "what are you waiting for, she is chocking". The attendees then started moving with fastness and retrieved a machine for this purpose. They guided the clear suction tube down her plugged throat. Esther had absolutely no gag reflex. This instrument was inserted into her inflamed throat and she never announced any apprehension. The continuation of the suction became useful and cleared Esther's blockage. Esther was taken to the Grimshaw Hospital by Ambulance for a period and then administered into the Peace River Hospital.

Once Esther arrived here in February of 2010 her stay would be endeavored for six months. Her residence would become a small room with the scent of disinfectant. White drapes, curtains and sheets were everywhere you glanced. Long curtains were pulled for privacy from strangers. The bathroom sink and toilet were stainless steel. These quarters were shared with a neighbor from the same room. Your closet was compact. Your single bed was dressed with starched sheets. They were recovered routinely. The humming and beeping sounds of machines called continually. You became one more human attending the continuous flow of hinder. The weak would surrender their bodies to Heaven. The others would struggle for absolution. New recruits would become members on this thing called life and death. The fear of being forgotten could weigh heavily on one's mind. The feeling of losing your identity was powerful. Your will would be tested and tried. Your ability to show resistance would surface if you were strong enough. Your determination would show others that an attempt was being made to not expire. The energy put into living one more day, made you a guest in this hospital for one more night. With time you adjust to the system of this new world but would not entirely become accustomed to their ways.

A STAY AT THE HOSPITAL

Ernie and Esther gladly accepted the invitation for supper. They had just pulled into town from there long trip to the city. Esther ate a small amount of food as her bowels hadn't expelled any material recently. She felt tightness in the chest area. Ernie naturally navigated towards the Grimshaw Hospital. If there was a slight chance she was having a Heart Attack he was pursuing his travels to get aid. Esther however did not have substantial pain in the heart region. This offensive heavy feeling seemed to interfere with her breathing. The detour made the arrival with Ernie announcing Esther's specifics. The staff quickly took precautions and attached her to heart monitors. They could guarantee Esther that the intense tests revealed that her heart was not the culprit. Her lazy bowels were making havoc on the rest of her body. The medicine Esther was digesting was and would cause severe constipation now and in the future. To live with this discomfort was torture. The length of this assault could not be determined. No mercy would be found to conquer the injustice placed upon her. Terrible Stool Softener could be added to your regular medicine practices. To manage and survive this grueling ordeal could happen. You did not have to plead for relief. With such distress Esther swallowed the softener with encouragement. It would work its magic after nine and a half stressful hours. This urge to vacate would attack the bowels with such force. She was ready to blow like a rocket. Esther would have to be prepared to occupy the restroom and settle for a while. In the future when Esther's dormant bowels became active all else stood still.

One last trip to Ontario was fulfilling Esther's thoughts. She presumed they required a much needed visit with Ernie's brother and family. They could reacquaint themselves with the nieces and nephew that had been strangers for far too long. This should be completed before any more health scares arose. Ernie realistically knew that a vacation would just prove to be chaotic. The unplanned quick trips to restrooms would be alarming for all involved. Keeping medication prepared for such an ordeal would be daunting. The strict routine that Esther had would be painstakingly frustrating to those unaware of her needs. Ernie could sympathize as he would also enjoy the company of his brother. He also knew Esther wanted to remain surrounded by family near and far. He would not be making this venture a possible one. Their health issues were just too complicated to over shadow. The strain and structure of this kind of undertaking would not be forgiving on both of the bodies. This wish of Esther's was not going to be granted.

AN OFFERING

Esther and Ernie made slow steps around the Grimshaw Cemetery. The plot that appealed to them was in the last row facing south. Esther would be informing the family as to its location. The rock that the twins had engraved should suffice as a head stone. Esther wishes to be cremated. She does not want a lot of money spent on her funeral. The service should be respectful. Those are her words of choice.

Ernie and Esther were on one of their usual drives. Smith Mills country by Dixionville was in their scope. The area reminded Esther of one Sunday when I was very young. Ernie and Esther piled all of us giddy girls into the big old station wagon car. We were in dire straits for some meat of any kind. The family was suffering due to low income coming forth. General Motors was on strike. This car dealership was Ernie's employer at this time. Ernie had driven up and down these rough dusty country roads over and over. There was nothing but nature to focus on. Not a wild thing in sight. Ernie was so hoping that a wild Deer or Moose would surrender himself to us. This particular Sunday there were many hunters on every strip of trail. Ernie was becoming so agitated with all the disturbances in sight. No smart and swift animal was going to step into a clearing with all this commotion going on. To make a deliberate shot with the rifle into the woods was not practical. The nervous hunters were impatient and touchy. There were no assaults made at all so far. The day continued without any real luck. Ernie drove the packed dirt roads with strained eyes. Gradually and with just slight notice a massive dark shadow became visible as it peacefully sauntered into view. The strong huge antlered Moose slowly with uneasiness continued to step forward onto the open cut line. Ernie quickly surveyed his surroundings. The area was strangely clear of all others. Even the woods had a quiet hush about them. Ernie proceeded to gather his nerves and the talented hunter stepped forward. He steadied his rifle and lined the gallant Moose in his sights. The wholesome animal reared his giant head and then bowed in approval. Without hesitation Ernie fired a deadly shot. The lifeless Moose had made the ultimate sacrifice. This offering was truly a blessing. Without notice the forest had soon produced hunters from all directions. The abundant noise was back again with more velocity. The forest was alive once more with the sounds of people. Ernie retrieved this sacrificial animal as quickly as possible and returned home a happy man.

DEAR FRIENDS DEATH

Esther had been the recipient of dismal news. Her dear friend had been diagnosed with Cancer. A deadly Tumor was invading her arm or shoulder and was intruding on her ever important liver. Her family would decide on Monday what kind of ruthless action would be taken. Esther new her family must be so shattered with the damaging information. Esther felt so much dismay for her suffering friend. Her tired colleague along with her husband had a vacation planned for Mexico. Esther could speculate that this disagreeable Cancer would put a halt to their plans.

Esther purchased a small white dog with black eyes at a gift store. The stuffed dog resembled her friend's poodle. The soft Teddy Bear had the initial K on it with rhinestones. Esther wanted her bewildered ill friend to know she was handy to help and possibly smooth her undeniable worry. Esther and a pal went to visit their declining feeble friend in the Grimshaw Hospital. The family knew Esther was confirmed to show as she had requested an appointment. Esther thought her dear friend was looking better than expected. She had however faltered a great deal in the last three weeks. Esther would cherish these simple but short times. Esther offered the Teddy Bear to her friend with sorrow. Esther had silently wished she had given her the small memento sooner. Maybe it slightly would have meant more as her friend was becoming confused with time. The Cancer patient had been placed on the Morphine drip now and oxygen was used often. The toxic Cancer had slithered and snaked through her entire body. The Cancer had invaded her veins, nerves, capillaries and blood vessels as their own road map for all directions taken. The doctor presumed that Christmas may come without her in it. A nice death to Esther was to endure no pain. She hoped and prayed that her friend would die with little suffering. Esther had her reasons for seeing her this one last time. The family now would have the fearful task of being witness to her conclusion. Esther couldn't handle seeing the sadness so close up. Esther did not want the glimpse of seeing her dearest friend go through the journey of death. She knew her own family would be going through their own crisis soon enough. Esther's own mortality was already staring at her through a tunnel of unexpectedness. She wished she could give more security to her friend but could not continue on her own path of living as she watched the uncertainty of her own life.

Friday the twenty seventh of December 2003 came and went. Esther's tormented friend was still clinging to life. On the fourth of February Esther's son in law got the chilling call that she had finally surrendered and withdrew from this life. Esther informed me with the latest and displayed a whimper in her voice. I had also at one time become very fond of Esther's friend. I had dated one of her sons. My time was spent with her temporarily. I could recall her sweetness towards me. I enjoyed her family very much and was gracious for their kindness. Esther and I cried openly as we were stripped of our defenses. How I wish I had been visible to give her suitable soothing embraces. I know this particular death was extremely hard on Esther. This was supposed to be the opposite way around. Her friend was to be attending Esther's funeral., Esther was to face death first. This puzzling mystery left her shaken and disturbed. Cancer was intolerable and so very cruel.

LONG TERM CARE

The recent study was complete. The Health Care System had requested Esther be sequestered into Long Term Care. Esther was now a resident of the Peace River Hospital. She should be placed with qualified nurses that would be able to handle her needs. However the Sutherland Nursing Home in Peace River had no vacancies. Esther was then administered as an outpatient in the regular ward of the hospital. She would remain in these quarters until a suitable room became available. Her care givers were put in an awkward position as Esther required continual care. The nursing staff was tending to many patients and were already running on fumes. Esther would feel guilty bothering them with her requests. Her issues could take up valuable time. Esther's comforts would have to be observed and dealt with. Esther was not put in this ward of her own accord. She just expected to be a resident of the nearby Nursing Home. The trained staff would be educated about her unique needs in this department. The enormous lack of long term housing needed to be rectified. Esther would only find strength and solace in her town limits. Health Care plays a huge roll in one's betterment.

Esther would have a hard plastic brace made for her lazy right leg. It would extend from her foot right up until the base of her knee. This would help support her small framed body. Her balance would be equalized more sufficiently. This might be a remedy for the slight drag she brings forward with her foot. The brace was strong and sure but a complete nuisance. It was more of a hindrance than a relief. When the brace was assembled we would be exhausted from the struggle. Esther would comply with the walking exercises as she felt a duty to use it once intact. Esther would glide herself along the narrow hallways with the assistance of the guard rails installed. She would not demonstrate too much independence. Esther was terrified that too much of an expedition could be reason for her to vacate the premises. Now that Esther was committed to the hospital she was adamant that her future was here.

MY MANY TRAVELS

My journeys to Grimshaw from Bonnyville have become many. The small highways are sketched in my memory. The scenery changes with the four seasons. The horizon stretches onward. The signs along the roadways show more mileage ahead. The pull offs are mine along with other travelers. Gas stops become familiar land marks. My friends live along these prairie roads. Their assistance if needed has given me peace of mind on these long stretches of pavement. The semi, logging trucks and oil rigs are more evident now than in the past. The vast popular oil industry has taken hold of the riches in our lands. The Derricks are placed along my journey to Grimshaw. The golden fields in fall are full of rusty colors. The hours pass by with solitude. I replace the quietness with loud tunes for which I hum. My senses intensify when I see the Great Valley coming into view. The hills are alive with rustic orange, yellow and red leaves. The mighty river flows with superb force. Down the noticeable curvy road etched into the soft hill I roam. When I surface on the other side of the Peace River bridge I know I am almost home.

MOMENTS WITH ESTHER

Arriving at the hospital made me eager to get Esther outdoors among the emerging life. This change of scenery was a welcome distraction. It would reawaken her sensitive limbs. The slow walker could make her manipulate her sleeping muscles. The wheelchair would help us manage Esther around the scenic hospital grounds. She could see the splendid view of the peace valley from here.

I would initiate the process to take Esther to her true home on many occasions. On this particular pass we would be recalling the autumn colors that were changing quickly. These days exposed her overloaded memory to much she wished she could replay over and over. We would witness her superb moments of splendor. We toured through the rolling hills of the Shaftsbury Trail, towards the Mackenzie Cairn Monument. The hills were vibrant with every kind of color imaginable. Leaves were just starting to lose moisture, which would produce the wonderful array of bronze colors. My purpose was to get Esther into the spectacular river valley. We were all touched by the beauty.

My next treat for Esther was a successful retreat at the valley Market Gardens. Esther's weakness was all vegetables, especially the green kind. Baby fresh peas were on my radar. To us the baby greens were like candy to our taste buds. I was so thankful to purchase the vegetarian chocolate. Esther so patiently waited in the hot car. It was extremely tiring for her to adjust to and from the unit. With my return, Esther occupied the front passenger seat. I placed myself in the back. With precise pressure I could force open the shell. I would energetically squeeze the firm pea pod. I then would gladly gift Esther with them. Esther could not muster up the weight that was required to puncture the pea shells. Her hand was becoming disorderly for such a task. Esther savored the flavor with each small pea that entered her month. Of course this was a rare treat from her usual.

We slowly maneuvered closer to the ranch hidden on the hill. We quietly positioned the car close to the barb wire fence. The horses with shiny coats and manes of straw like hair were housed here. The friendly mammals came gingerly up to my hands that offered green succulent grass for them to graze on. They enjoyed our company. Esther would have instantly wanted to rub that soft spot between their nostrils. The smile on her face was from sheer gratitude. Esther and I got to equally absorb the moment with the mild mannered animals. The small crease lines at the corner of her mouth were made of true jubilation.

We continued on our quest to the popular Bear Lake Rodeo grounds and campsite. We had spent many sociable hours on these sparkling waters through the years. We had all with excitement handed over an abundance of money at the annual midway that would pass through town. The Rodeo mastered all the favorite events. The Chuck wagons brought out the little gambler in all of us. This weekend was a few days we all looked forward to. The small town would house strangers. A large crowd was a welcome sight. We enjoyed the change immensely. In 1977 or so Queen Elizabeth of England made an appearance at Bear Lake. With her attendance being of great stature, they changed the name of the lake to Lac Cardinal. The area had the fortunate luck of getting many upgrades due to her visit. This handy place was and still is the center of many town functions and attractions.

Our perfect busy day was sure to end with a tasty meal. We dealt with the heaviness of the wheel chair. We glided Esther with precision into the home through the tight doors. Supper was then eaten with vigor. The dirty dishes were on their way to completion. It was essential for Esther to use the nearby walker, as she would navigate her way around the spacious kitchen. Ernie and I were in conversation. Esther was to my back. Literally a second went by with the two of us in translation. With sudden movement I caught Esther in my vision. She had lost connection with the sturdy walker. Before I could react, Esther's body was toppling to the kitchen floor. Her head made contact with the hard surface of the linoleum. Esther thought she would be able to judge the distance from the handy walker to the stainless steel sink.

Esther was in mid motion when her body became rigid and she just stopped. Esther lost her stance and tumbled straight backwards. Her delicate head and solid floor made a crashing connection. Her fragile skull actually bounced up and down with the gravity in action. Ernie and I were weakened with complete shock. My dreaded thought was that she had broken and stripped the use of her neck. She was so privileged to rise up and stand beside us. I couldn't fathom the thought of her shaken on my watch. Ernie and I would have been wrecked with guilt. Esther was just performing a task she had completed so many times before. This manner of balance was not capable of producing her brains requests.

REALITY SUCKS

Esther's visits would soon become less frequent. She was finding visiting her home brought on a multitude of friction in her heart. Coming home periodically teased her wants. If she were to flee, the damage wouldn't hurt so much. The sure energy it took to shift and transform the body was draining. Ernie and Esther would be drenched with perspiration. I believe Esther had to gravitate towards peace at this time. Some inner comfort would have to be mastered here. She knew it was time to escape the grips of the world that was once hers.

The flowers Ernie had so lovingly planted would not be hers to tend. The green grass that would start to creep through the moist earth would not be felt under her sensitive feet. The chirp of baby Robins in the tall willowing trees would navigate flying without grace. The birds would be taught to surf the sky with or without her presence. The promise of a hot summer night's shower would be produced in the high sky. The thunder and lightning shows would go on regardless of who was in attendance.

This huge yard held so many years of wonder and the happiest of times. The fenced in area had seen its share of tragedy at its hardest also. These memories would become just that, demolished with time. Esther's children, grandchildren and great grandchildren would make new traditions of their own. They would learn to treasure some of her teachings and others would be forgotten or replaced with their own ways. Her life as she knew it was truly now in the hands of God. She was not coming home to live anymore. She was retiring to the hospital to die a certain death.

HOSPITAL LIFE

Esther would be moved three times in the regular wing of the hospital. The rooms were just temporary stops. Finally after three strenuous months, she was delighted to occupy a private room in the Long Term Care Wing. This was really just another block within the regular hospital that they had named Palliative Care. Esther would now commence payment of certain fees to be a patient in this wing. We would arrange to have permanent TV and phone setup as an addition to her new lodging. She was so pleased to have her own personal room. The privacy would be accepted whole heartedly. Her personal belongings could now be placed without the worry of invading the space of others. Her small area was hers alone to personalize. The big window made the view extra special. The Peace River Valley entered your view and captured your sight. The picturesque scenery helped with the days of control loss. With three months behind her, Esther had learnt the new ways.

The girls were making their routines ritualistic. The welcoming staff at the Peace River Hospital was familiar with their appearances. The second eldest daughter would begin the present day with her appearance. She worked in the valley. The senior daughter had employment at the hospital so she was on permanent stand by at all times. My twin sister would make a daily entrance at Esther's room. Ernie functioned with continuing his important aid in Esther's wellbeing. He would gather at Esther's room in the early morning. He would commute back for five o'clock supper. Ernie would excuse himself with the darkness of night.

Esther's trips to the airy cafeteria became a huge delight. The eating room was spacious with an entire wall capturing reflections in the clear glass. A communal vegetable garden was on display for all to see. Witnessing the growth of that produce was a joy for all. Many among them could not participate in the successful harvest that was evident. Ending at the basement level for a simple tasteful coffee meant a moment of freedom. Escaping the pale room changed the monotony of her long stretched days.

Her hours consisted of regular medication. Meals would be opposed by her mighty looks. Bowel movements took effect if she was to be lady luck today. Restful naps were taken under the watchful eye of the passing nurses. A pleasurable shower would excite Esther once a week.

Esther would try to engage herself in written material. Her changing eye sight was a challenge. We would supply her with any large word enhancing device we could get our hands on. Kobo would have been the perfect tool for Esther. She could have read the large print with clearness. The frustration she experienced with loss of sight would have been minimized.

Some hours would pass quickly with friendly visitors

making clever conversation. Her son in law would graciously meet Esther on Sunday mornings for their usual round of cards. She would redeem her title as skillful and cunning victor. It gave Esther a chance to use her wisdom that was awakened with the challenge of cards. She could ponder strategy and divulge her wits when necessary.

Esther was extremely lucky in deed. She had love pouring out of buckets from her family and close friends. Many other patients consumed their time strictly alone. No eager company would stop by for conversation. No laughter or tears were heard from other spaces. Many were placed here and then soon forgotten. It hurt my aching heart to see some fade into the white walls. Esther was presumably the envy of many residents. Esther had the attention that many craved for. Her room usually consisted of company. The patients and staff could observe the affection we showed her daily. Esther was handed a rough sentence, which she had to endure every living day. She was also blessed to have volumes of love on a grand scale. Many wish for this thing called love and never get to achieve it. Esther was floating in it.

TUMOR ON THE MOVE

After Esther completed four months in the Peace River Hospital her Brain was striving to do more damage now. Her increasingly shrinking body weight was of grave concern. Esther's right hand was now just about completely paralyzed. Her right leg had become so rigid and useless. Her sensitive teeth were tender and sore.

As the Brain Tumor became more hostile it affected her sight drastically. Her eye prescription had failed tremendously. Esther was forced to retire almost completely from reading. She became so desperate to focus. She was adamant about having an eye operation. It was impossible to change Esther's mind. She was making plans for the improvement of her inadequate eyes. Her Dentist and Optometrist were the ones to make the intelligent choices. Leaving nothing to chance we quickly and urgently placed a call to her professionals. We couldn't justify making appointments with them. We knew what was to be reported and stated. Esther was at the mercy of her enlarged Brain Tumor. She was a member of a small town which accounted for the personal setting. Both her doctors were a married couple and practiced in their individual fields. They were familiar with Esther's unique situation. They relayed to the family that they would sympathetically go speak to Esther in person at her private room. With straight forwardness the team considered Esther's case and simply could not initiate any procedures on her at this stage of her disease. They did not want to make Esther any empty promises. With great patience and tenderness the doctors put Esther's struggles into perspective. They truly felt her despair and left broken hearted. This couple of professionals put their businesses on hold so they could adhere to Esther's calls. That was selfless and commendable. They were so wonderful with her and eased our dread if not hers. The family would try to console Esther as her expectations were becoming dismal. Her issues were spirited now and we were all unclear about the future.

Esther's twin daughter that lived in Grimshaw was a Hairdresser by trade. The Sutherland Nursing Home was attached to the hospital. They received permission to use their beauty room. Esther was in need of a hair makeover badly. A perm would relax her unruly doo. Being on constant medication and having her major operation had left Esther's hair to thinning. With purpose we wanted to achieve some normalcy for her. The drab would leave and she could accept some delight with her new curls. Esther got situated at the wash basin to have her hair rinsed. Her daughter was using tender practices learned to extend the neck into the steel basin. She could not get Esther's head to cooperate. Her neck would not allow the head to bend properly. She certainly could not use forcible pressure on the powerful neck. This would cause undo pain and possible damage. Every position was manipulated with no success in sight. Esther's head would not yield forward or backward. The necessary angle could not be achieved. Esther's daughter was wasted and whipped. Esther was pissed and pestered. The extent of the happiness we wanted for her literally went down the drain. There would be no repeats of today.

BABY FOOD

Esther was requiring her meals to be pureed. She hopefully would not choke on the smashed food. A large visible note requesting this task be completed was placed by her bedside. Esther's gag reflex was not permitting any solid foods to enter the mouth and then be swallowed. Esther had occupied this area for five months now. She would still often receive her food as solids which in no way could she ingest. Esther could not accept her pills if not crushed like dry black Earth. Again routinely her medication was dispensed to her in hard shaped powder.

She was encouraged to swallow a protein drink that had the consistency of condensed milk. It was incredibly thick like molasses. At meal time this substance was exchanged with her normal intakes of calcium. This lard like spread would attach to her white teeth. The drool produced would drip from the corners of her mouth. She could not tolerate the strain that was produced at the entrance of her soft lips. She would sacrifice and take the risk of blocking her airways. She preferred the white runny milk immensely.

We along with Esther would get frustrated with these easy little mishaps that were not being noticed. She would regrettably and reluctantly have to interrupt a busy tense nurse. This meant accepting whatever fate was returned with an already over worked person. Esther would try to be prepared to handle the consequences that came along with her intrusion.

No moisture for your circular pills meant the entry of no pain medication. It was all relevant. One couldn't happen without the other. Her imperfect meal would become cool along with the extra wait. Esther's army would inject at moments when no relief from pain was seen without a reminder. Esther's inner mouth would get so parched. A cotton ball shoved down inside her voice box was a good description. The urgency for water soaked her dry throat.

LACK OF CONTROL

More moisture would produce more urination. During the lonely evenings her bladder would almost explode with readiness. She would reluctantly push her buzzer to disturb the needed nurse on shift. Whoever responded would have to quickly intervene and rush Esther to the awaiting washroom. This urge to urinate was becoming more and more frequent. Esther and the staff on hand were finding this situation impossible to master any longer. Esther required her moisture through fluids. To keep up with the constant release of her urine was certainly a burden. With great defeat, Esther had obliged to wearing adult diapers to bed at night. To rebel against the usage of these was pointless. Esther was being sentenced because of her untamed organs. The questionable Depends made more sense. This dryness would improve the length of her slumber. The worry of notifying the nurses was bound to happen less often. With her continual decline came the ultimate execution. Esther was placed with the nuisance of a Catheter. All points of privacy were now extinguished. Her private parts were not so anymore. The attached tubes would assist Esther in the release of her inner fluids. The plastic bag could hold huge degrees of liquids. This ultimately accommodated all involved with Esther's wellbeing. The Catheter became a part of Esther. The benefits of this Catheter became a source of ease. The advantages improved all of our anxieties. The Catheter was easy to empty and handle. Even Esther was relieved at its usefulness. The delicate location of this device would make Esther prone to Bladder Infections however. It would be dealt with promptly and would clear with proper attention.

RED STRAWBERRIES

Esther's appearance was showing clear signs of weight loss. It was apparent that her appetite for bland hospital food was becoming nonexistent. Esther would slowly with apprehension uncover her food tray. She would with irritation quickly cover it up again. She would try to smother out the lingering smells. The colorless sight of food would make her stomach roll with protest.

Ernie became so determined and desperate to feed Esther. We were on a mission to find our own food grinder. We purchased a small one and immediately put it to work at Ernie's home. We pureed Esther's favorite fruit. Bright Red Strawberries pulsed out juice for the tasting. That evening for supper Esther was delighted to witness the change. She inhaled the sweet Strawberries. She relished the tasty morsels. They glided down her throat with ease. She was so touched to have tasteful and colorful food to eat. Ernie would from that precise moment on glad fully bring Esther delicious fruit. Esther was so blessed to have Ernie present to relieve and soothe her hunger. Ernie felt purposeful doing this small little task for Esther. This taste was a welcome distraction from the usual here.

A NOTICABLE VACANCY

Ernie's life had been altered tremendously. He nursed his ill wife through the long days and nights. She departed their home. Esther was placed in the hospital in a quick moment. He barely had time to take a deep breath. A complete change of life had taken place right before his worried and exhausted eyes. Everything at home had become so quiet and vaguely normal. The house was drained of sound. The activity was at a halt. The habits of the days past could be neglected. The automatic reflexes could rest awhile. The stillness was needed. The calmness was granted. Ernie required a well-deserved rest period. During this down time he would be facing the truth. Ernie and Esther had been stripped of their unity. Having Esther in an environment where she could be cared for properly was Ernie's main goal. He was strangely perplexed about his feelings. Esther would manage better in her new surroundings. The large, four level spilt home just didn't feel right without her presence. The aroma of Esther preparing succulent meals in their spacious kitchen was gone. The variation of flowers growing and stretching for the sun didn't seem so pretty after all. The continual upkeep of the house just seemed mundane and pointless. The visitors stopped making appearances with Esther's absence. The girls found their childhood home a place of sadness. The four walls that contained Ernie and Esther's belongings could in reality all be replaced. The sentimental value of ones treasures get measured when you don't occupy them any longer. My secret haven and place for sanctuary suddenly became a place of my past.

Ernie's days of caring for Esther were changing. He now would complete the twenty minute stretch to the Peace River Hospital. This was enforced two or three times a day. Ernie would carefully spoon feed Esther her meals. Smooth strides glided from the generic plate to her awaiting mouth. Esther could not consume anymore rations. Her hunger could be satisfied so easily now. Her loss of appetite was all too common. Her small frame had been reduced over the last couple of months. Her petite figure was shrinking.

ERNIE AND ESTHER'S UNION

Ernie and Esther looked forward to their simple times of togetherness in the cafeteria on the lower level. It became a need to satisfy their times of boredom. Family and friends could concentrate on worldly matters away from her hospital room. She was not the center of attention here. It was pleasant to hear news of someone else's life. To be a part of the functioning population for a time was pacifying. We all took to the coffee shop for normalcy. To be away from the hectic pace of Cancer was accepted. A smile could even be produced in these surroundings. It made the sadness bearable. Cheerful thoughts would present themselves.

The midafternoons were spent with Esther and Ernie resting their weary eyes. Ernie would get comfortable in the portable rocking chair I had purchased for him. Esther would stare at Ernie while he snored in the corner with the sunshine resting on his face. This quiet time would make her ponder about her tainted disease. She would try at all costs to keep her depression at bay. She regrettably would wonder about Ernie's future without her. She would really try to focus on the present and not on the inevitable distance.

Esther would cry over her debilitating pain. Her frustration over people not understanding her ordeal would cause her grief. Through all of her uncomfortable commotion she never issued the words, "why me".

Esther seemed to understand that it could always be so much worse. She had experienced much happiness and sorrow in her life. Esther was extremely grateful for family and the friendships she had made. She invited a new day in every morning and strived to see each one as a true blessing.

Ernie would arouse for his ritualistic morning coffee with his male friends at the Grimshaw Hotel. The other local customers Ernie would also greet with light heartedness. He could escape from all the wrongs that were following him. He could pretend that all was right in the world. He became relieved of his worries if only for a short while. The camaraderie of his fellow buddies supplied him with balance. A watchful eye was always present. All knew what was transpiring in Ernie's circle. To be widowed was already facing many of Ernie's friends. They had already been through the steps of grieving. They would be patient and steady for Ernie.

Ernie's nights were filled with trickery. The finality of Esther's absence built up unclear visions in his thoughts. His vulnerabilities would surface when he closed his eyes. Esther's departure from the home built a surplus of anxiety. Most dark nights for Ernie were enveloped with distant sounds. Esther ringing her little bell was a typical occurrence. He would rush the stairs to check on her. Reality would come forward and make its self-known.

The opposite was rare and welcomed. Relaxing dreams would enter his sleep and supply him many hours of rest.

His severe stiffness would not show mercy however. His aching back would plague him and not show any signs of weakness. His sore bones would stretch as he exited the couch. Many five a.m. early mornings would find Ernie filling his thermos with rich hot chocolate. He would enter his truck when the rest of the town was hushed of movement. Ernie would do his regular tour around the lake. He would find a peaceful spot off the main road. He would ignite his heated seats with a cup of coco and lose himself in silence. The comfort of the truck seats along with their heat made the pains subside slightly. Ernie's early escapes would find him visiting the weigh scales. Finally he would continue onto the hotel. He would make an appearance once the rest of the world was awake and present.

BEGINNING OF THE END

The beginning of Esther's long awaited end started on July Twenty Eighth, 2010. Ernie lazily entered my twin sister's flowery back yard. She was relaxing on her sunny deck. She had just finished mowing her thick growing grass. My oldest sister had placed a call of distress. She relayed the message. Esther had been feeling ill this particular morning. Esther could not find the strength to raise her head from the hospital beds mattress. Her neck muscles could not support or balance the weight of her head. For the last month or so we had noticed her head had started to tip slightly to the left. Esther without much grace but sure determination was attempting to nourish herself. She had succeeded in applying the soft mush to her entire face and her clothing. The progression of the slightest bit of meal sliding down her angled throat was a cause for chocking.

The enlarged Tumor of Cancer is being intrusive and invasive. The Tumor is now attacking all sensitive parts of her body. The controls of her inner and outer shell are going to be challenged soon. The force of the disease will be noticed and felt.

Ernie proceeded to the hospital at around one thirty p.m. My twin sister was in transit to meet at Esther's room. Mild activity had filled Esther's day. A discussion took place with the family members in attendance. Should Esther have a companion accompany her through the night? Esther conveyed her annoyance. She wanted no extra treatment placed on her. She would be perfectly fine.

Esther utilized her hospital room all the following day. She had a total lack of desire to make a switch from one place to another, or from one position to another. To justify the act of motion escaped her. Esther would have preferred absolutely anything compared to wasting valuable time in bed. This sense of worry was creeping into her thoughts. She could not tolerate this uneasiness she felt.

Esther was complaining that her left side was irritable. She was experiencing soreness and tenderness in her hip area. The nursing staff would carefully place hot compresses on her delicate side. Hopefully this would aid in her suffering. When the intense heat would not suffice the cold compress was given a try.

CLEANSING THE BODY

Thursday July 29, 2010, my twin sister arrived at the hospital about ten a.m. Esther has been confined to her bed. She did however try to consume some of her breakfast. Esther stated to my sister that she needed to go to the washroom. Esther had been taking stool softeners to help with her episodes of constipation. Mild Diarrhea was much gentler on her system. Esther was trying to stall though and control her urge for a bowel movement. There was a male nurse on duty. Esther really just didn't feel comfortable with him having to witness her much needed stool release from her body. Esther finally just could not wait. She literally was going to burst if she lingered any longer. They quickly called the staff to assist Esther to the washroom. A new nurse emerged. Esther is a bit nervous. This new lady she has not encountered before. Esther's movement has been absolutely rendered; she must now be placed in a portable device that will support her slender frame to the bathroom. This unit transfers the weight from the nurses to this strong movable aid. This way the nurses don't have to physically exert themselves while moving her. This contraption looks horrible and terrifying to my sister. It reminded her of what maybe a butcher uses when hanging meat. The nurse gets Esther prepared to be strategically arranged into the awaiting lift. The very moment the lady begins to lift Esther's filled body; the direct pressure on her protruding stomach begins to make havoc. Esther cannot stop the raging bowel movement. The escaping stool is running out of her panicked body like a slow moving creek. It is messing the white crisp sheets on the bed. Droplets of brownish poop follow her and are making a trail from the bed to the toilet. Esther is understandably upset. This is so completely embarrassing to her. What can she do but watch in disgust as her body neglects to cooperate? The staff gently place Esther on the white porcelain cold toilet. My sister has placed herself on the edge of a nearby chair. She is ready and waiting to intervene if she must. She so wants to be by Esther's side. The small space only allows so many bodies. So she waits dedicated not to leave. My sister is intensely watching Esther be tolerable of her condition through the open door. Esther asks my sister with unease in her voice to "please don't leave me." My sister can see the worry in Esther's dulled scared eyes. Is Esther speculating that this is the beginning of the end? Does the human body cleanse itself for what is to come? Esther does not have to convey what she is feeling; my sister can see the dismay on her face. Esther keeps complete eye contact with my sister. She constantly wants reassurance that my sister has not disappeared. A wonderful, kind and special woman comes to help in the room. This nurse assists with the capable lift once more. The awaiting stool was temporally on hold until the pressure made contact. They repeated the process back to the white throne. Esther verbalized that she thinks she is done for. Esther is not adjusting well to any of this commotion. Esther is slowly starting to have perspiration gather on her body. Her breathing has become labored and tense. She can taste the threat of nausea entering the bottoms of her throat. Esther is so drained and spent with exasperation. The energy it has taken from her well used form can no longer fight the beast raging inside her. My sister will always recall the desperation in her defenseless eyes. The very gentle nurse whispers to my sister "when is Ernie coming down?" My sister states that he would be making an appearance later in the day. In a gentle but direct tone the nurse suggests that my sister notify Ernie to come as soon as possible. Ernie of course without hesitation arrived promptly along with my eldest sister.

Esther was discouraged. The day was spent in bed once again. To bring up and brighten her mood we casually mentioned that maybe she was due for her regular coffee break later. Esther looked so forward to those simple spent moments. It was difficult at this time too not want to make her wishes come true.

The professionals proceeded with chest and side X-rays. This became a horribly long stretch for her. The pain in her side was starting to become extreme. It was not in Esther's character to state how it was becoming unbearable. The nurse administered morphine by a needle dispenser in her right hand. This is Esther's bad arm that is basically paralyzed. They chose to leave her left hand mobile so she could still use it if necessary.

EVERYTHING PUT IN ITS PLACE

The nurse on duty suggested we meet with the Doctor in the afternoon to discuss Esther's future. All were in attendance except for me and my second eldest sister. She was on holidays. The doctor believes that Esther's Tumor has now grown to the point where it is going to completely cut off her breathing. Her head won't stay straight because of the Tumor growing in size. She more than likely will develop pneumonia. It already sounds like she has fluid in her strained lungs. Esther was told twelve years ago, when diagnosed that she would eventually choke to death from this fatal Brain Tumor.

Esther signed a Level of Intervention Order a while ago. This stated that no measures were to be taken to prolong her life. Level three meant support and comfort only. This meant no feeding tubes, no antibiotics for infection, no CPR or treatment to support life. Only pain medication could be administered to be made suitably comfortable. Each of Esther's girls and Ernie had a copy of this Order at our homes. If Esther was ever to be present at our residences and she should have a mishap that would cause her to collapse, the order would be shown to the appropriate Medical Professionals on hand. They would at this time not produce any life savings measures.

My twin sister has no doubts that this is Esther's last week of life. She said she doesn't know why, just has a feeling and has seen such a drastic change in her progress in these last two weeks. She has noticed clues, such as her body getting rid of its waste, her neck refusing to bend properly, Morphine for pain and not getting out of bed for days.

The family that was present for the meeting with the Doctor slowly pace back to Esther's room. I am sure Esther must sense the concern the doctors, nurses and family feel about the progression of her failing health. The sisters have made direct, true and serious calls to their children. The girls start to mention to Esther that the grand children that are situated close to Peace River will be making unscheduled visits. Esther should be seen while she is still able to converse with them. Things could go sour very quickly and any last minute regrets should not be taken. The time to see her is now.

My twin sister has polished Esther's perfect nails over the six months she has been present at the Peace River Hospital. Esther would request her manicures be completed on the weekend. She found the long days of summer occupied everyone's valuable time. Saturday and Sunday stretched without visitors. Everyone had duties and chores that had to be completed. These sorts of things were usually left for the weekends to tend to. It was pleasant for Esther when my sister would arrive in the later week. My sister just cut and filed her strong nails this particular time. Esther had depleted her energy for her signature pink polish this week. Her nails on her right hand would dig into her palm as the hand was in a continual ball for a year. She could open the right hand now only with assistance.

July Thirtieth, 2010 surfaced with Ernie and my twin sister arriving at the hospital with their protective shields up. My eldest sister also made a planned stop to visit Esther at ten a.m. Esther does with great difficulty try to force herself to swallow the breakfast which has been made for her. Her day will be extremely long as her condition does not seem to be getting any better with time. Esther still is requesting Ernie to produce the succulent strawberries for supper tonight. That tasteful fruit she looks so forward to. She however will not be able to eat or drink as she had planned. This purposeful action of accepting nourishment and fluids has all but stopped since this morning. Her body is not producing any moisture for her organs. Her mouth has become so dry and unbearable. Esther sucks on soft pink foam that is dipped in water. This warm fluid soothes her constant unpleasant deficiency.

ESTHER'S VOICE

Esther's doctor makes the awaited appearance in Esther's room. Ernie is so relieved to see him as questions need to be answered. The doctor reviews Esther's file. He knows her extremely well and has witnessed her struggle from the very beginning. Esther, ever so direct and with complete control says to the tall, slender doctor, "so this is the end, I am dying?" The doctor stares straight into Esther's brown glassy eyes and with the same directness states "no one can know for sure." Esther says with gallant calmness, "I am ready and tired of this fight." The doctor seems to be searching deep within himself and his soul, as he is quiet for a very long moment. His knowledgeable eyes scan our faces with grave concern. The doctor with quiet sureness makes mention that he will issue morphine by the drip now. This should control any of Esther's pain that she is experiencing. It can be administered every two hours by a family member. I without hesitation made way for this task to become mine. I solely took on the role of giving Esther the strong sedating Morphine. I knew the girls already had their roles to play in Esther's wellbeing. I wanted this duty to make absolutely sure that not one drop of that powerful medication was missed. Esther would not feel any unnecessary pain as long as I was at the controls. The strong Morphine drip would soon bring solace and peace to Esther's small framed body. By the end of today, all of Esther and Ernie's daughters surrounded them like protectors of the Holy Grail. With calmness and support for one another we would be Esther and Ernie's Army once again in the face of uncertainness. We have requested no visitor's at this point. A sign has been placed on Esther's door stating as much. Absolutely no one was getting into Esther's room without our permission. On this particular day Esther had several people wanting to visit. Simply put, we just mentioned that today was a difficult one and please come back at another time. We would also keep a watchful eye out on Ernie as he was just as frail right now as Esther.

A HOME OF COMFORT

The long stressful day ended. I proceeded to remain with Ernie at my childhood home. I just felt this intense desire and need to take care of him. Esther was under the watchful eye of the other girls. They had so lovingly and purposely directed their energy towards Esther's wellbeing. Ernie required someone to watch over him tonight. I was going to be his invisible guardian. I could sense his big guard of amour was being shaken to his core. I would keep him in my vision and always just a glance away.

Ernie and I talked slightly as the darkness filled the living room. We were both exhausted so we knew it was time we turned in. Ernie slept on his usual couch. His back would be placed up against the backboard. He seemed to find comfort there like nowhere else. His grandchildren's favorite sleeping bag would creep up to his chin and keep him toasty warm through his restless night ahead. Many confused dreams would sweep and creep into Ernie's thoughts.

I slept in Ernie and Esther's vacant bed room that evening. This space had not had occupants for months now. I had the most peaceful feeling laying there under the many blankets that were soft and warm. The lingering smell of them was present in this space. Total comfort and easiness surrounded me like a giant quilt. I truly felt like a small child again. All of the world's troubles and pain could not touch me here. All the safety I felt was surrounding me like a glow. I was truly in complete and utter bliss just having their soul's surface to touch me. The spirits from my grand childhood gathered and sent me soaring through memories long forgotten. I had loved entering this big bed when I was a young girl. When my parents would leave for a night out, my twin sister and I would purposely fill their bed with our little bodies. We felt secure and safe. When Ernie and Esther would arrive home, Ernie would gently and carefully place us into our own beds for the remainder of the night. These true life treasures are what my foundation as a person was built on. Be kind and caring to others but stand your ground. Work hard and enjoy your rewards. Be responsible for your actions and don't blame others for your mistakes. All the basic fundamentals were taught to us in this spacious house that was enveloping me on this very special evening. I was so truly blessed to absorb all the sensory emotions that captivated me tonight. I may never have the chance to be a participant in that pleasure again. Deep within my mind I accept this fulfillment as a gift. I am sure that this home of comfort will without warning disappear from my grasps.

PALLITIVE CARE

Saturday July Thirty First, 2010 is filled with unsteady emotions. The nurses have been so kind and generous and very thoughtful of our dilemma. They watch the family come and go, back and forth, as if we are lost and searching for something that we cannot find. The moments are becoming guessing games with Esther's progress. Ernie is spending so many long stretched out hours here at the hospital. My twin sister has made the portable rocking chair as comfortable as can be. Hopefully this will tend to ease his pains which he is experiencing with standing for long periods.

The nursing staff have detailed to us that the Palliative Care Room is now available should we want to move Esther from her present area. Once the name of this place is spoken, I now know that Esther's time is running out. The Palliative Room of course is only occupied by patients that are dying. Esther would like to see the option she has for a transfer. For Esther to see this spacious room is a challenge. To place her small fragile frame in a wheelchair is just too physically draining. Her body just cannot compete with the stressful situation. The trained and dedicated staff just focuses on pushing Esther in her movable bed. The awaiting room is only a couple of doors down. Esther in the past has put forth that she would possibly like this accommodation nearing her end. There certainly is sufficient space for a family to congregate. The patient's awaiting bed is at the far end from the entrance. The couches, TV, sinks, microwave and such are directly by the doorway. It makes complete sense to have the bed at the opposite end of this area. This way the patient won't be disturbed. The flow of people coming and going would be constant and could cause confusion for the patient. The adequate attention should be given to Esther while she would be the regular in this room. I wonder if too much activity would partake in the entrance area. Then I noticed that there was no TV for the patient. In this particular case Esther had become very reliant on this device. It had become her company, her companion, her distraction from all that consumed her. We have been instructed by the staff, for Esther to locate into this area she would require twenty four hour care from her loved ones. There would have to be continual care at all times. This is a huge commitment to make for everyone involved. Esther's Army would have to take into consideration many factors. Many jobs would be at stake. Families and lives would be altered during this state. The family consult over this new found information and try to see it clearly from all angles. Esther grants us freedom. She really just wants to stay in her small hospital room that has become her temporary home. Soon we make an appearance back in her private quarters. She is once again settled. Esther automatically puts on her tiny white earphones. They connect to the volume of the little black T.V. set she has placed directly in front of her. She without notice vanishes into her private world. She does not want to hear any discussion about estimation and time frames. She will cope and connect with her hidden inner strength. Her little device called a TV has become her security blanket. The noise she hears drowns out the worry and awareness she knows that accompanies this journey. She calculates her precious time is running out. She just wants to get on with it and let's go. But only one man knows for sure when her demise will end and he is not telling.

THE WORDS I MUST SAY

Esther and I are alone in her still and quiet room. I need to take this opportunity to tell her what she has meant to me. I may miss this chance. I need to channel my deep and emotional nerves right now. I strain my unstable voice and force out the words she must hear. I cry out of necessity. My eyes find Esther's. She seems so calm almost. The Morphine drip has made her very limp, lethargic and numb. I spit out my clear message and say "how terribly much I am going to miss you and you are the bravest person I know." She whispers back to me with, "really." She accepts my statement. She starts to say, " the tears won't come." She never explains anything more about her lack of sentiment. I never could ask her why? Her lack of energy, loss of fluids and medicine surely play apart in this. I hold her beautiful soft hand in mine. I know that I must not take this precious moment for granted. I sniffle and she blankly and directly states, "I can't cry". I love this woman so totally. I want to freeze frame every second now before the strong intoxicating Morphine takes her to a place I cannot go. The family rotates shifts with Esther and we each find our own peace within those four walls.

MORPHINE

The nursing staff has introduced Esther's Morphine site from her paralyzed right hand to her stronger left hand. She has also had this needle invade her flesh on her sore side along with her shoulder. The nurses don't have to inform us. We figure it out. Her slender veins are stripped and shutting down. Fluids must be present in a human's body for one to thrive. Esther's organism has been barren of moisture for some time. She is unprotected and defenseless against the malicious Cancer. Esther's lungs are intolerant to the substances entering there. Her breathing becomes labored. A congested sound escapes from her chest. The pain plagued in her side is so mean. The Morphine drip is continually administered. Esther still does not grumble or moan much. This is good news. This means the pain medication is working and doing its job. Esther will soon drift into a continual faze of unconsciousness. She has very few lucid moments now. Her mouth has not closed since her continual slumber came into effect. Her tongue looks like leather. She is producing no saliva at all. We take turns wetting her parched mouth with the moist sponges. She does seem to show the sucking motion. Her reflexes might be still showing some small action.

The day has become a complete blur. The nursing staff has been so tolerant and let us do our thing. We travel in and out of Esther's room like we are in a march of some kind. We have infringed on the visitors lounge with frequent use. The handy kitchen has been used effectively. Esther's presence has also affected the staff. Esther has drifted and breezed into the lives of her care givers. The nurses have gotten to see the most private of her moments. They have witnessed her sheer frustration, envy from a glance, spiteful anger and sadness so bleak just like us. They have also been privy to her smiles so sweet, her courage and persistence so mighty and her robust attention. But Esther's bright light is starting to fade. We are all starting to fuel our bodies with feelings of anxious tension. The minutes and hours are torturous on our souls.

LAST RIGHTS

My eldest sister questions Ernie about bringing in a Reverend to bless Esther. Esther found faith and worship comforting. She attended church regularly. She was a permanent fixture of the church. She belonged to the choir, Sunday school, prepared meals, teas and participated in every aspect when possible. Ernie is not particularly fond of attending church. He has never truly enjoyed listening to preaching and blessed ceremonies. Ernie's mother was a very spiritual woman and occupied the Anglican Church on a regular basis. She was a contributing factor for the churches existence. Ernie accepts that Esther would want this rite of passage to make her final journey complete. Ernie and I choose to exit while Esther is being tended to. My personal faith is very present and abiding today. I know the righteous powers will honor Esther. The three Grimshaw daughters are all in attendance by Esther's side. The Reverend enters Esther's room softly and commences her sayings with the truth she believes in. She is a small tender looking lady. She is very kind and does not pressure anyone. Her praying is direct and short lived. A little silent prayer is stated. The making of a cross is placed on Esther's forehead with holy water. The Reverend has disappeared as quickly as she appeared.

PURIFY

For hours now Esther's body has taken every breath with so much will. Her chest cavity becomes caved in with the continued struggle. Except for her breaths Esther's tiny physique is not with motion. Her shiny flesh is completely covered with a blend of odor and sweat. She forces the oxygen into her lungs. This act brings the limited air down through her clogged chest. This takes all her power to exhale. Her heart will continue the fight to thrive even if the body wants to surrender. The will to survive is stronger than the will to die. The nurses suggest Esther adhere to a needed sponge bath. Her fatigued torso is ridden of her wet night gown. Everyone leaves the stale room except for me. Esther is completely at their will as she cannot move or speak. The nurses cleanse her the best they can. They flip her immobile body from one side to another. They purify her tender skin. Soft soothing baby powder is rubbed into her crevasses and cavities. All this sanitizing makes me feel some comfort and ease. A new hospital garment has been replaced. I do however sense that this particular cleaning is somehow different from all the others. Esther cannot feel or smell the scent of sweet powder. This bath is as much for her as it is for me. This will be her last proper examination. The gentle nurses want to prepare her body for what is to come. The lovely ladies showed much remarkable compassion under the circumstances. Esther was given back her dignity and once more became a woman, mother, wife, daughter and a child of God.

ONE LAST BREATH

The long spent day has brought us to six thirty p.m. on August Third, 2010. We are all starting to feel the lack of nourishment in our bellies. Ernie and I are reflecting in the visitor's lounge. Two hospital meals have so generously been given to us. I accepted these meals with thanks. I could not muster the desire and will to eat mine. I would make sure Ernie tried to force some nutrition down. My goal in mind was to keep Ernie fed and on his own medicinal schedule. It was easy to fall and become withdrawn when feelings of sadness took over. I was devoted to being Ernie's self-appointed on call guardian. It was my privilege to stand beside him through this flawed time. His wellbeing and health was a major concern. Ernie's ample hunger met the food given with gratitude. My sisters were absolutely going to take care of any arising situations while we collected our thoughts. They had dealt with matters pertaining to Ernie and Esther all these years. Today's lows would be no different. The eldest daughters were going to go gather downstairs to the Cafeteria to see what they could force their mouths to swallow. My twin sister was sitting by Esther's bed alone. Esther's breathing has changed slightly. Her labored breaths were now longer and deeper but further apart. My sister's intuition was telling her that the time of complete rest was very soon upon us. My sister is holding Esther's frail hand and kindly saying, "it is ok to go, you have fought a strong fight, like a warrior". She drills these words forward, "we will care for Ernie and that is a promise." I believe those simple but important words were heard by Esther. Our vigilance is what she so desperately needed to go forward. Esther inhaled one very long labored breath. She held it for several seconds and finely and slowly exhaled. She took another struggled breath of little oxygen just like the one before. With no doubt in my sister's focused mind, she knew this was the coming final end. My twin sister with clarity called me on her ready cell phone. She was not about to leave Esther's side to rush to get us. She abruptly told me and Ernie to stride to the room this instant. She also simultaneously called the older sisters to retrieve immediately. Ernie quickly and quietly placed himself in a chair next to Esther. He neared her right side by her soft beautiful face. With no movement in Esther's body, he held her tiny hand in his calloused one. It was only a few short everlasting moments and Esther blew out her last flickering flame. Six fifty p.m. was Esther's time of demise. Esther's internal energy was now empty. She was already making her departure and proceeding on and up to the skies above. I stood motionless and paralyzed on the opposite of Esther's bed. I was staring blankly down towards her noticeable frigid body. I was suddenly mystified by what my eyes were capturing. Esther's facial features were morphing into skeleton like colors. Her face became extremely gaunt and dim. Her apparent looks however did not frighten me. They were

233

recognizable from when my Grandfather had parted. Then with sudden quickness a soft warm glow was forcing its way through Esther's form. A white dimensionless cloud like misty substance was flowing ever so slowly around her. A presence underneath Esther was raising her gently and carefully towards the ceiling. Esther and this apparition became one all its own. I was totally focused on this essence right now and not Esther. This transparent free moving wonder was only for my eyes to see. Esther was exiting this world for another. Esther was becoming one more soul that would meet the father, the son and the Holy Ghost. Her existence was leaving her carcass. It all vanished within seconds. The transformation was complete and ended before it began. The shaken older girls entered the hushed room. My twin sister and I inched to the back of the somber place. They now had the overwhelming feeling of sadness enter their cores. The tear drops were raining from our eyes. Ernie's shoulders sagged. His guard wavered. His mask of protector became lowered. His shield gave way to emotions of pure sorrow. His aged eyes were lost and empty. Our beloved Esther was really truly gone.

My second eldest sister had made Esther a gallant promise before she died. Esther wanted upon her passing to have her mouth closed before rig mortise set in. Esther had been present and seen to many cold bodies with their mouths stretched open in distaste and it bothered her a great deal. My sister worked with many patients that had and would meet their maker. It was not uncommon for my sister to have requests of all sorts from her clients. She did agree to meet Esther's request. She did this noble task for Esther. She quickly and nervously closed Esther's mouth. She also tipped her head slightly until her body hardened.

The twelve years had finally come to a conclusion. We all sat in total disbelief. There was no action from anyone. We justifiably were in complete and utter shock. We had seen in the future this day coming over and over. It was here and now we were not sure how to handle the loss. My brain and body were drenched. I was not capable of any sudden changes. The anger, guilt, frustration were all taking up space in my mind. I could however find solace in the fact that Esther was a true survivor of Cancer. She embodied the word completely. The execution of her death surrounded me with relief. Esther was granted entrance into a world of sure joy and happiness I hope. I was so truly thankful that any of Esther's suffering was suppressed and now vanished. I had sincerely hoped that I had prayed enough to make a difference. Had God heard me over the years? All I sincerely wanted was for the family to find some peace in a world so powerful with doubt and helplessness. We as a unit were all stripped of our contentment. Necessity was conquered and exercised for Esther for twelve years. Our nerves and emotions were raw. We would need some time to mend our broken hearts. Our senses needed to be rewired. Our hardened shells would become soft with time. Smiles of joy and laughter were a pleasure we missed. But now our large cries continued as our own bodies were becoming haggard and drained. Ten lingering minutes vanished before we called for a nurse to make our assumptions correct. The nurse had no doubts. She forces her words of regret out, "Esther indeed has passed away." The family would be granted time to grip the reality of the sight around us. Esther lied so still in that single white bed. I kept waiting to hear some kind of sign from the heavens. Shouldn't choirs be singing, skies of dark clearing over head? It was so final so fast. After all this time I expected more, but more of what I wasn't sure. My final good bye was spoken from a distance. Esther had her family rallied around her at this time. I was satisfied that Esther had heard my words of love previously.

Esther continued to occupy the mattress on the shiny metal bed. Her death was surrounding us. We urgently needed to vacate this oxygen less space quickly. The family beforehand had decided that once Esther's passing was complete we would clear her room speedily. This removal was to be achieved suddenly. To come back tomorrow was a chore no one wanted to face. We had all spent many downcast hours in this small square room. To enter without Esther's presence would be shattering. We secured all her belonging in boxes and bags. This collecting of her treasures was strangely sacred. Her tiny watch, numerous glasses, diamond earrings were gathered, handled and protected with the utmost care. This process of packing while Esther lies there now seems very distasteful to me. I watch the others do this task through blurred vision. I am in a fog and not sure that I am doing anything productive. I seem to be standing motionless. My wandering eyes glance to Esther often. Barely time has passed when I realize that I see Esther's flesh is certainly changing. Her soft clear skin is taking on the discoloration of a very bad bruise. The variety of colors startles me. She is developing the hue of pale yellow mustard. Then a tired green like a plant that wilts without moisture. I wanted to recall Esther's beautiful clear and glowing face with clarity. I could not be present to see the display of dark and dreary colors for one more second. My time in this place was over. I had to escape. The lack of precious air was sucking me in like a vacuum. I exit quietly and closed the heavy door. I stationed myself in the doorway corner. I was to shaken to move any farther. A nurse on duty saw me struggling with my composure. She took me in her gentle arms and held me tightly. She hugged me and held me near. We both cried our tears of pain and sorrow. This caring nurse was also a friend of mine. She felt the loss and sadness. Her kindness and sudden empathy was much appreciated that day.

The many vehicles were packed with mementos of Esther's existence. The family all ventured to Ernie's to take comfort in familiar surroundings. Everyone had left late into the night. Ernie was finally resting with much needed withdrawal. My twin sister and I proceeded to my parent's room to sample some rest. It was awkward for my sister as she felt uncomfortable in their bed. I on the other hand could have slept there for an entirety. We both placed our over sensitized bodies on the firm mattress. My sister went to adjust and move her body slightly for better placement. As she did the mattress somehow slid slightly off the frame. We dare not wake Ernie for his assistance. He required his much needed rest. The pressures of the past days had made us stupid with laughter. Our giggles eased some hurt away. Maybe Esther was playing a joke on us. That would have been like her. My sister and I would continue to talk way into the early morning. Finally fatigue would win and sleep would take over. My sister would not sleep without discomfort. The obvious slant in the mattress was slightly annoying.

THOUGHTFULNESS

Ernie and I would not venture far from his large house. I guessed family, friends and acquaintances would be bringing food made with love and kindness. Gorgeous flower arrangements would enter the house. The sympathy that was being shown was so overwhelming. Over the next couple of days the continual drop off of flowers came in every color, shape and smell. The weather was so very accepting that many vases were left outside to enjoy the warm sun. My sisters were on a continual basis receiving and accepting bouquets just for them from their close friends and such.

With all this warmth flowing around the house I became slightly jealous of all this attention going elsewhere. I had a weak moment of selfishness. I felt quite silly and tense. I looked at my other self being my sister and said with dumbness, "none of these positively beautiful arrangements are intended for just me." My sisters were receiving so many directly intended acts of kindness. I also wanted that feeling. I had arrived alone in Grimshaw. I did not have my family or any close friends here by my side. Even though Grimshaw felt like my home and my sincere feelings for my old friends had never wavered, I guess it had just faded away. I had been gone too many years. I was just a familiar face to many. The realization was that time erases all things permanent or not.

CHANGES AND CHALLENGES

My world had become a constant moving vessel for years. Had I stayed anywhere long enough to really make an impact on anyone's vision of me? All the years of travel with small children in tow had made me guarded to making friendships. The lack of trying meant no one got their emotions hurt when I left, especially me. I am not tolerant to goodbyes. My sensitive side always surfaces and then the tears of sadness come. It became my practice to make sure the children's inner self's were complete and satisfied. It became the same ritual at every place we encountered. A new town meant new surroundings and new people to figure out. A game I got quit tired of actually. My sense of stability was always on edge waiting to be notified of another change.

The uneasy motions of moving had stopped finally in Westlock. We lived there happily for seven years. The children embarked on their early school years there. We had grounded true close friendships. These superb men, women and children became very special to my heart. But the world does not hold promises. Working for others always puts your ethics on the line. When that doesn't mesh well then it becomes time to relocate again.

The choice was Banff or Bonnyville. You would think scenic Banff would level higher on the acceptance scale. "Not", too expensive, too far from family and my husband just didn't fit the code there. He gave it his all but just couldn't see himself working in this environment. He never really got the chance to make good contacts and lasting relationships working at the Mountain Lodge. The type of people he was meeting were transits just passing through. My husband was in the business of building strong and fertile partnerships with members of the community. His calling was seeing the old men every day in for morning coffee. The business men you shot the shit every day. This atmosphere was just not for him.

Off to Bonnyville we went. Fourteen years later we are still here. Children are finished school and finding their own ways in this strange but fascinating world. They have become the strong individuals I look up too. They show kindness caring and generosity to others. They expect nothing in return. They also have made mistakes and errors along the way. Their choices sometimes have had huge consequences. They have dealt with their insecurities and paved way for each other. With gladness in my heart they have bloomed into something wonderful. They have worked hard and played harder sometimes. They are strong in their beliefs and stand by them. They are sensitive to issues that mean something to them and represent that. They are my pride and joy every single day. The one thing that I know for certain that I have done right is make kind hearted individuals. I am certain without them my world would not have the sparkle and shine that it does.

But moving to Bonnyville was not an easy adjustment for any of us. We all left extremely tight and secure friendships. Having the camaraderie of those people was missed greatly. To have to place my worried and confused children in new schools was terrifying for me if not for them. My husband and I were fortunate enough never to have to experience this new adjustment at an early age. We attended the same school through all the twelve years.

I also began the promise I had made to Esther. Smoking was extinguished from my life. The elimination of Nicotine in my system was a road treaded lightly. This had to be accomplished now. Esther had to witness this while she was alive. My husband would have to put the new venture at Bonnyville on hold for a small period. A routine Pap exam was showing signs of possible cancer. The surgery to remove my Uterus and complete a partial Hysterectomy was rectified as soon as possible. My husband would pacify me for one week. He then loaded up and went to Bonnyville to start his new job as General Manager at the Bonnyville Neighbourhood Inn. I still had weeks to heal from my surgery. I would gently tackle all duties left to me with my husband gone. The great distance now between me and my family was huge. The drive to Grimshaw was going to take seven lengthy hours only one way. The worries of all the people closest to me were pulling on my frazzled nerves. I was not finding any real reasons to be happy here. I wanted my old life back. To be pleasant to others was a real try on my part. I did love life. I just at this point had a bad taste about mine. I was without a doubt going through some sort of adjustment issues. I could not find contentment. My happiness was shallow and lost. It wasn't any ones fault. I just felt alone and lonely. The combination of all factors was playing with my emotions. The move, quitting smoking, Hysterectomy, parents poor health and distance became a giant chore. It took me a lot of painstaking hours, days and months to come to some sort of terms with my misplaced peace.

ESTHER'S WISHES

The family searched everywhere we could think of to find Esther's wishes upon her death. This struck me as peculiar and strange. Esther would have without a doubt wanted these requests fulfilled. Many of us new bits and pieces to her plans suggested. Ernie along with us all was none the wiser. The words of her wishes should have been placed right where her important documents were always secured. We eventually found a box with some minor proposals mentioned but nothing more. Ernie did not even have a guess for us to search. More clarity should have been made prior to her death. Maybe Esther never did any more than what we found. Near the end possibly she found that in the big picture of things these were not as important as once thought. Four years after Esther's passing my twin sister came across some papers of Ernie's. While Esther was in the Edmonton Hospital she had indeed made Ernie write down her valuable wants. In a bundle of notes were the words clear and profound. With so much confusion at Esther's early diagnosis Ernie filed them away. We came across these special words when Ernie was moving into an unassisted living house in Grimshaw.

I stayed with Ernie during these days of him granting permission to proper individuals with matters pertaining to Esther. Ernie was so over whelmed with all the commitments to appointments. Planning and completing funeral arrangements was heartbreaking. Legal matters were tended to and could be complicating. Banking institutions had to be notified and dealt with promptly. I tried to make Ernie focus on the present tasks at hand. I was eager to keep him nourished, full of pleasant thoughts and keep his company coming. I was so worried he would fall into a state of depression. His whole world had changed over a course of days. He had been so full of daily regiments with Esther. I was concerned that because the rituals had come to a halt he would become stifled. After all the dictation was complete and tended to, concerned visitors stopped making appearances, the house would become silent. What would Ernie see as important now? He would have so much free time available. He hopefully would not become broken and crushed. The future for Ernie was up in the air like a balloon and I was wondering when it might pop.

After Esther's initial death her body was delivered from the hospital to the Memorial Home in Peace River. Esther had chosen to be cremated. She wanted her ashes to be present at the service. Esther also wished to be escorted to the Crematorium by someone she knew, meaning a family member or a very close friend. She wanted this assigned person to be physically present in the vehicle that was touring her body to be cremated. She had been fearful that her body would actually disappear or be exchanged for another during this travel. She wanted to be guaranteed absolutely that no mistakes during this trip to Grand Prairie could happen. My twin sister's husband was very comforting to all, as he volunteered to literally drive Esther personally to the building in question. He also had been his own father's guide back from British Columbia to Alberta for his funeral. He would be Esther's chauffer. My other brother in law came forward as well and offered his services to accompany Esther to be cremated.

Now that the journey to Grande Prairie was set in motion a suitable body casing had to be chosen for Esther's final expedition. All four girls along with Ernie entered the casing room with silence. There were shiny elegant Urns on display. These Urns came in all different shapes, colors and price tags. Some of these pieces of art were modestly priced at several hundred dollars. Others were in a league of their own, with thousands of dollars advertised on the ticket price. The actual wooden boxes were in the same room but on a different wall. These were made from the richest of woods to the fire kindling used outdoors. Ernie had a major decision to make. Esther had to be transported to Grande Prairie in an appropriate box with her son in laws. The cheapest wooden box was very practical. Esther would be strictly going from the wooden box in the van to the awaiting embers in the burning chamber. Ernie would do circles in his head of which was the correct decision. He did not want Esther to actually accommodate a pine box; she was too good for that. A middle of the road casket at four hundred dollars would suffice.

Esther would surely desire to be clothed in her favorite flannel pajamas along with her fuzzy slippers. Her special crotchet blanket that she always placed on her lap to keep her legs warm went inside the coffin too. Her older sister had made the little square blanket that Esther cherished and took everywhere. A small detailed Native American doll that was dressed in the proper attire was to be placed close to Esther's body. The coffin was now complete with all of Esther's treasured items.

AN URN FOR ESTHER

Ernie and the girls had in conversation the previous day come to a conclusion that one of Esther's metal Tea containers would be perfect for Esther's ashes to be held in following the Crematorium. On the way out of the Memorial Homes casing room, Ernie and I were the last ones to exit. As we slowly walked past the Urns in their display cases I mentioned to Ernie how lovely some of the etching was on them. I had never seen a real Urn before. Ernie and I were mesmerized by their beauty. The more we stared the more I could see Ernie was deliberating the difference between an appealing Urn and an old Tea container. Ernie had a change of heart and wanted Esther placed in a safe, secure and completely shut Urn. Both of us entered the occupied room with the girls. Ernie voiced his decision and made it known that he was leaning on purchasing an Urn for Esther. Ernie and I staggered back into the casing room one final time. We deliberately made time to search over all the different types and sizes and materials these Urns were made of. Ernie had found one that he thought was appropriate. It was very strong and made from marble. It was a purplish color and in the shape of a rectangle. This Urn would stand the test of time. It would not disintegrate with the weathers hard snowfalls and windy days of summer. This piece of hard, delicately designed marble was six hundred dollars. Ernie was satisfied with the outcome and was more at peace knowing Esther was well taken care of.

As there was a few moments at the Funeral home where all were just pacing in different directions waiting on the boys to finalize all matters pertaining to Esther's journey. I could hear them just on the other side of these wooden doors. Just as I was about to enter through them a man came and did just the same and startled me. I realized that I had just seen Esther's wooden coffin stretched out on a gurney. It was put to the side for the time being. I knew only her body lied there and not her spirit but I still wanted to go to her. All I had to really do was place one foot in front of the other and walk up to her. I was so close to striding through those double doors and seeing her one last time. Just as I was to make my planned move I saw the casket enter the back of the minivan. My chance had been shut down. Probably for the best.

Once these matters were dealt with the trip to Grand Prairie could commence. These two men found the inner strength to guide Esther into an awaiting van. The front of the casket was literally only feet from them. They both entered the spacious van. One placed himself behind the wheel while the other was on stand by for whatever might occur. They finalized Esther's important wish. I know that she sure was very proud and honored to have these men at her side. This is a task not done by the men of weak. Only strong and compassionate people can complete this ritual. They made her trip complete without the worry that she so desperately feared. On that day all of Esther's son in laws except one would be with her on her travels to another dimension. My sister's husbands should know how much that meant to me and her. I did not want her to be alone; they all stepped up without concern for themselves, just plain love for her. Who would have thought Esther was the one that had a hold of their hearts all along? She had so simply touched the men in her life with constant care and wisdom. My eldest sister along with her husband followed behind the van. My sister pushed the button that entered Esther into an oven of heated finality and into the eternal flame of glory. She wanted to be present and complete this last act of devotion for our Esther.

The Funeral Home detailed the requested service sheets with speed and practice. Ernie picked out a glorious picture of Esther to accommodate the front. Her peaceful and content self was situated in front of her layered flower garden. The red poppies gathered strong above her in the back ground. Her prized possessions were enveloping her frame with purpose. She seemed at peace at home surrounded by her many flowers, the colors of the rainbow.

My niece designed a unique centerpiece to be put on the headstone at the graveyard site. This was made with weaved pieces of wood and crafted veins. The grand children were instructed to each place something that always brought Esther into their minds. The spray was enveloped with an assortment of memorabilia. There was a stick of gum still in its wrapper. Esther would hardly ever give you a whole piece of gum even though she had plenty to share. Her peeve was to see people chewing their gum like cows chewing their cud. Esther's signature pink lipstick in its green marble case was also placed amongst the many. The Queen of Hearts was inserted in the spray to commemorate the love of cards she had. Elephants of any size, color or make was Esther's absolute favorite. Why or how Esther got the desire to collect Elephants is not really known. Maybe she always wanted to see them in their own habitat in Africa as she loved to travel. Lottery Tickets were some of her pleasurable time dissolvers. Esther somehow always found the energy to enter various contests. She entered these random draws from Newspapers, Magazines and stores. She became very lucky on many occasions. She won a grand prize of ten thousand dollars once from the store called Super A in Grimshaw. I remember Ernie calling me with the news that they had just won some big money, of course I called, "bull shit." Esther's favorite things all became a part of this unique master piece. The lovely spray was indeed a sight to see and was made solely with complete love and admiration the grandchildren had for their Grandma.

Two of the middle aged grandchildren took it upon

themselves to make a collage of Esther for the hall entrance so everyone could grasp the tender and yet strong woman she was. Esther could be as soft as a rose pedal or as stubborn as a mule. Either way made her who she was and we loved her indeed for every quirk that was her. The plastered pictures were of her as a small child living out of her log home back in the Valley. Some were of Esther with a young tall and handsome man named Ernie. Many of these pictures had Esther with her children, growing along the way. Others were with her church friends and Multiple Sclerosis mates and just her everyday coffee friends. The collage was made with sweet devotion and looked beautiful.

SERVICE DETAILS

The family all gathered at the Royal Canadian Legion. It was time to put the hall into some kind of arrangement and order for the future friends and family that would be arriving for the service tomorrow. Two large tables were situated at the front of the hall. One table was covered with the large Quilt that her four daughters had given Ernie and Esther for their Fortieth Wedding Anniversary. Two pictures of Esther were enlarged and placed in black photo holders. A baseball bat and glove were placed on the table showing that the sport was dear to her heart. Antiques were a large part of Esther's life. She had books describing values of coins and glass of color and old china. She dutifully kept on top of prices of today and yesterday. The spray was up front and center and people were encouraged to take a look at it after the service. With the distance of the seats it was hard to really fathom the sprays entirety. You had to be at close range to really get the personal attachment to it. Long rectangle tables were centered at the back of the hall for the guests to mingle and show signs of friendship and understanding. Chairs were placed in two rows down the length of the hall for the service to take place. I made sure to put Kleenex packages on each row. I knew people would lose their composure and show their weakness through tears. This way all of Esther's friends and family would not be caught off guard without any eye or nose wipes. When the hall was looking complete, we could all take a breath of relief. Tomorrow would be the hardest day yet. To really let Esther go was going to be so damn hard.

As we were all just pacing for a moment, I noticed a very familiar face enter the hall in the distance. It did not take me long to have my arms wrapped around him in a choke hold. This was a very old friend of mine that I had not seen in years. He just wanted to come by and give his regards to the family. I think in that moment he was not really sure how to handle me strangling him. I guess, when I saw him, and I had no one of my own, like my husband or kids around, I just grabbed him because he was such a trusted and kind friend to me and I felt really lost and he gave me comfort even if he didn't know it. I am kind of embarrassed about it now but at the time it was what I needed to get through to the next day.

That evening we all surrounded the patio at Ernie's place. I was studying Ernie with great interest and concern. Ernie was carefully and intently taking the bottom off of Esther's Urn. With extreme care and gentleness he was placing some very small colorful rocks in the Urn with Esther's Ashes. Esther treasured a collection of rocks she had gathered over the years. We all regarded Ernie with soft stares and easy words, so as not to put Ernie under pressure. When his task was complete, Ernie secured the lid on the Urn with very strong glue. Ernie was taking extra measures to guarantee the closure was void of any extra air that would cause moisture and mold. Ernie was having a moment of dire need to keep Esther safe and warm from external elements. I took Ernie aside and just simply said, "Ernie, you know we don't have to put the Urn in the ground. Esther can stay in the Urn at home with you. It can be placed in your plot later or never, the choice is yours. Just realize that there is no right or wrong way to do this process". The thought had never really occurred to me until that very second. Esther even though in an Urn didn't have to be buried. This is exactly what Ernie was wrestling with inside his being. In the end he just couldn't put her in the cold dark ground. He just could not let Esther go. Ernie passed his decision onto the family. The Reverend would just mention that at the service, there would be no burial.

FAMILY FROM ONTARIO

Ernie's brother unfortunately would not be able to attend the funeral with his wife. His two daughters and one of their husbands would travel the long distance from Ontario to be with us. The eldest daughter was less of a stranger. She had visited over the years with her father and mother. She is such a special person, she portrays comfort and makes you feel warm and at home around her. I had not physically been in the presence of the other sister for about thirty five years. When I was a lanky teenager, she was a beautiful goddess of the same age. I was a small town gal and she was brought up in the big city. My sister and I, we wished to be just like our wonderful cousin someday. So many years had passed, that when I had to go on to the Hotel to greet them properly, I was excited to see how much we had all changed. As we were pulling up to the hotel I noticed a male and female having a cigarette in the designated area. I absolutely without a doubt new with in an instant that this gorgeous girl was my cousin the stranger. I hugged her and it felt like an old friend had returned from a very long journey. She was familiar and similar to both me and my twin sister. It was so right to have them there and be supportive of their extended Haas family. I was so grateful that the three of them had made such an effort to be there for all of us at this unpleasant time. Their mother was a very special lady that was a close friend to Esther. She was married to Ernie's brother. It was a complete and utter shock when three short months after Esther's passing, we received a saddening call. Their mother had also passed and was another angel among many. It has made me ponder the question that maybe destiny was involved in their deaths. Their close friendship could continue just in another part of the atmosphere. They would have each other for comfort. They will be watching and waiting to guide the next individual. Can't wait to see it, the two of them being the welcoming committee into Heaven?

SAYING GOODBYE

Tomorrow was upon us, August seventh at one p.m. The families all appeared at the Legion Hall with dread on our minds and heavy sorrow in our hearts. We exited the waiting vehicles and with a steady pace forced our heavy feet to the front of the hall entrance. Many sad and lowered faces greeted ours as we continued through the small entrance into the quiet waiting room. All the appropriate and immediate family members were circled around each other. My particular family would have to endure this service without my physical closeness. Richard would be there for our children and assist them in any way he could, but today Ernie had my whole attention. Ernie would be entering the main hall with me on his left arm and my twin sister would be on his right side. I was not prepared to let Ernie walk down that long isle by himself. The Haas family entered the big space and took our allotted seats. I could not let my own health problems interfere with today's issues. Ernie was very passive on the outside right know but that could change in any moment. I spotted a tassel on his pale green pants. I started to twist and do loops with that strand of material for the entire service. To lose my sanity just for a moment would mean total loss of control. If I really gave in to what I was feeling being glued to the chair that I desperately wanted to exit, my composure would be terminated. If that was to happen I may never recover for a long period of time so it was imperative that I stay focused and steady for Ernie.

The Reverend's passages from the bible were passing through my ears but I don't recognize a single word. It's like I have cotton stuffed in my head and is full of mumbles. However I got the internal feeling that what she stated was holy and true. I so wanted to be present in mind, body and soul but new my own difficulties were waiting in the wings to take over. I tuned into Ernie and just blanked out all the rest. All the girls had their attending husbands and children in tow, but up until this point I was without any of my immediate family for tenderness. Ernie and I had been the loners of the family circle. I stuffed the emotion of loss and loneliness in the back of my thought process. I only had Ernie on my radar. I was not crying, more just little tiny bursts of sighs through the service. I was wondering why? Everyone around me was full of continual sniffs and sobs. I was so numb with doubt and lost in the sorrow that was over flowing in that giant room. I had to be brave for Ernie. My tears would fall greatly through the endless days of sadness that were to come.

Esther Charlotte Marie Haas was born May Fourteenth, 1940 – August Third, 2010. Esther was seventy years of age. Esther attended her service; her stunning purple marble Urn was placed in the front of the hall for all to see. Esther's Eulogists both gave words of compliments and conscious displays of her values and beliefs and her true passions and loves of life. My brother in law and my second eldest sister dealt with the memories with control and strength. A personal passage from the bible was completed by another dear friend. Celtic music was played throughout the hall; we thought the sounds were reminiscent of the Scots. Esther's heritage was Scottish and English. Esther requested that the songs, Those Were the Days, What a Beautiful World and Will You Remember Me be played. The program stated that only family and close friends were to continue on to the Grimshaw Cemetery for the burial of the Urn. When the service was completed the Reverend made a mild correction, there would be no burial at this point so everyone was encouraged to stay at the hall for further fellowship.

I must mention that during the whole process of the service at the hall until the supposed burial. A wonderful holy spirit was with Esther the whole step of the way. One of Esther bride's maids had not been able to arrange it so that she could attend Esther's day. This lady truly has a heart of gold. She had gotten one red rose, it was to be placed on Esther's Urn for the duration of the day, and was not to leave that spot. This dear friend did not want Esther to travel this journey alone. She wanted to make sure she was there for Esther s exit. This true commitment and continual friendship and the passion she felt for Esther was a blessing for all of us. We knew she was not riding solo.

The funeral service had come to a final end. The family was to exit the hall and commence back in the holding room. My son gathered Esther's Urn in his safe sure arms, and brought her back into the room awaiting. Eric was Ernie and Esther's only grandson. This special closeness of today would be Eric's duty. We took Ernie's arm and with utter dismay filed through the line of weary eyes and dismal facial features from the many people that had attended. For some strange reason all this finality hit me and I let out a whale of a sound from my throat that I just could not contain anymore. Once we all entered the room I found my children and made sure that they were handling this very new adjustment of sadness. They looked somewhat lost and very grim. This was something very foreign to my children. Very few funerals had they been witness to. My husband was in the hall catering to guests. I was Ernie's shadow. My children were handling the hurt and pain extremely well for me.

The reception was complete with the usual finger sandwiches, desserts and cold and hot beverages. It was heartwarming to know that Esther and Ernie and family had so many well-wishers handy. To see familiar faces that were also not seen on a regular basis was comforting. Everyone soon was to leave the hall, but they were sure to give hugs and let us now that we were all in their prayers and thoughts.

Esther and Ernie's immediate family were all

requested to continue over to my sister's house for more tasty food and relaxed visiting. It was very reassuring to see Esther's family gather together. I kept thinking how much Esther would have enjoyed talking with each and every one. My sister put much effort into making them all feel welcome in her home and in her beautiful yard. The weather was so warm that we actually sat in the shade of some big trees that offered shelter from the hot sun. My sister put on another delicious meal that her husband BBQ. There were kids playing on the green grassed hill which was just behind the house. The dogs were chasing each other for fun. When the animals were all played out they would go for much required attention. They would lie at our feet to be pampered. Everyone had their bellies full of good food and good beer one more time. The conversations between all had memories replayed in our minds, some humorous, sad and all together were times we would truly never forget. The day had been a long one. Goodbyes, with hugs and words of solace were presented from all. I hate goodbyes and would rather say, "See you next time," this doesn't seem so final and pressured. It might be a stretch until I see these faces again. Our chances and circumstances of meeting again will hopefully be seen with much joy instead of sorrow.

GOING ON

From this point on I occupied a basement room at my twin sister's home. I did not with good conscience forgo my stay at Ernie's home. I knew I would have to eventually make my way back to Bonnyville. I missed my children and husband more and more with each passing day. Ernie would regrettably have to start to live with in the walls of his home as a single dweller. I guess I had to let Ernie go. I knew the impact and the extreme anxiety would most certainly occur. The fears of a new life alone would unleash feelings and make Ernie confront the absolute terror that we had predicted would surface. Lonely days and nights would creep in the door at Ernie's house. The girls of course would be present at every moment that Ernie needed them. Their arms of comfort for hugs and their warm words of encouragement would let him find extreme peace at his own pace.

I finally returned to my home in Bonnyville after being gone for one stretched out month. My family greeted me with tender hugs and sweet kisses. How I had missed the loving arms and happy smiles of my two beautiful children. My husband was patient and strong when I needed him to be. He showed me caring and love. Our unity and perseverance with yet another obstacle had survived to greet another day in this crazy thing called life. We had tackled this abundant storm with conscious strength and undivided companionship. We made it through to see clear skies on the other side. More hard blows would surely come our way, as this is what life delivers, pleasure and pain.

Now that I was home where I could relax and unwind my grief had become so much more real and forceful. I had been suppressing Esther's death for way to long and when it hit me, it erupted like a volcano. The red hot pain was so strong in my twisted gut. The pure love I had for this woman was vandalized and I felt every impact possible. My sadness had been growing with speed. Every night I would close my swollen eyes and would visualize her beautiful face. The deep love I felt for her would hurt so badly. The wetness would drip from my eyes as I would rock myself to sleep. I thought about her last days often. How could a woman so full of goodness and strength, a caring nature and a giving sole be handed such a devastating blow in life. We constantly hear that we should live our life to the fullest. Never take it for granted and accomplish all that you can. You never know when your time is up. That all sounds good in theory. If you can't walk to the starting line, cannot swallow that succulent food or control your own body functions, it really is just a crap shoot, and that saying goes down the drain. You can live the life you want when you are healthy. If you're mind works and your body works, everything is possible. I never once expected Esther to tell me she had one to five years to live because of a fatal Brain Tumor. By the way I will be spending my remainder of existence having radiation therapy, being nauseated, losing my eyesight, hair and mobility. She was only seventy when she died but lived the previous twelve years trying to out beat Cancer. I have felt bitterness with the world and have felt cheated and defeated at certain times. When she breathed her last breathe my life changed forever.

CANCER SURVIVOR

That was then and this is now. Esther never surrendered to the disease of Cancer. She fought harder than anyone. She did it with grace, strength and the utmost courage. My tears now are to cleanse my soul and heart. I want to portray Esther as a true Cancer survivor. She beat the unfavorable odds. She found a prevalent solution that made her unique body last another gracious seven years. She must have found her own fountain of youth deep within her mind. Her positive attitude steered her in the right direction. Her Army never let her down and was by her side continuously. Esther had the support and backbone of her loved ones standing tall when she would bend slightly. I only cry now because time was passed to quick, but I got to spend twelve incredible years with the wonder woman that I had undying love for. Everyday really was a precious gift. I did eventually lose my Esther. I try not to make the world that is full of pain and bitterness turn me hard. I cannot see Esther in life but deep in my heart I let her linger and wonder on. I know that Esther waits for me in the next world with all the ones I have lost before. I know Esther and God are all right with each other. Esther was needed elsewhere and I think she would be ok with that. Remembering the memories bring smiles and tears. Forgetting is worrying that she will slip from the minds of others.

MIRACLES

I love you mom. It is an honor to be called one of your children. I will figure out a way to get through this uncertainty I have to battle within. Learning to conquer my own fears can be challenging. With the family as a team we will always try to look for the light that is you shining through the darkness .We will continue to just keep moving forward and do what will need to be done as life unfolds for all of us. Your absence in my life is felt every day and I miss you terribly. A part of you burns in my heart.

There are two things I know to be true in this life. The first thing is that without any uncertainty that Ernie will have a grand place in heaven for him when he vacates this universe. Ernie did more than his fair share of capturing Esther's disease called Cancer. He pounded it into the ground until there was no more room for escape. His perseverance and continual guidance just never exited his being through this whole ordeal. Saints I believe come in all shapes and sizes and Ernie was Esther's private saint here on earth. The second thing is that Esther was truly a living miracle. She was not supposed to exist after five years with this burden. She lasted the five and another seven more years with the Brain Tumor. I have seen what having faith in the human spirit can accomplish. When we as a whole can work together and build bridges for the less fortunate, we can give someone the courage, strength, and determination to face death or any obstacle with grace, dignity and strength. Most of us will never have to face what Esther had to deal with every day for twelve years. To not be able to control your destiny must be very frightening. Esther thankfully had a family that rallied around her like mountain so high that no other obstacles could enter her circle of protection. That barrier we formed never thinned for 4380 days. We all sacrificed, so she could concentrate daily on continuing another grueling yet successful day. When we had to lean on each other, we did so because we all new that at the end was survival.

SISTERLY LOVE

We had many conflicts and battles with each other as sisters. Our quarrels made us encounter intense and powerful brawls. Four women could bring on turbulent and passionate contention. Our attacks were brought on by frustration and circumstances beyond ones control. We however in the end always came out showing appreciation for the other. We would find a balance that worked for us. We all went on a difficult journey. We experienced extreme sadness but also were privileged by being witness to Esther's beauty for life. We stayed with each other until Esther's end. Each one of us specialized in a certain area over the others. Our talents were used accordingly. Those twelve years fighting for Esther make me tremble with the thought of how we also survived Cancer.

My sisters will truly never understand how much I cherish them. Being the only family member that had moved away for decades has the tendency to make you wish you could be a part of the closeness the others get to share day by day. My heart longed to be with them but distance has a way of robbing you of the changing dynamic. So now I have a perfect opportunity and chance to let you know my sentiments. We are all so different in special ways. I am proud of everything we have all accomplished. Your children and mine shine through our eyes. Everyone is special and unique in their own precious way. I wish all the absolute best to each and every one in my family near or far. All our girls are strong, vocal independent women. We had a great teacher in Esther. My boy is kind and always pleasant and has the temperament of a sunny day but can show strength like a storm waiting to burst. In other words all our children are like sugar and spice, a perfect mixture of sweet and saucy. They turned out just the way they are supposed to. Polished and ready for whatever comes their way. I will be on guard for you or them always. I am blessed to have you all in my life.

ACCEPTANCE

With the time that has past I am better with Esther's departure. I still cry often for I miss her. But now I can smile soon after because of the women she was and the wonderful testament she has left for me to explore. She left me with many great memories to wipe out the bad. I sleep with one of her small square quilts under my pillow every night. This is a small way for me to still feel her presence. I know the fabric is touched with every bit of her. A favorite picture of Ernie and Esther stare at me from the wall directly across from my bed. Every night with gratitude I still get to say goodnight to my two favorite people in the world.

With Grimshaw so far away I have also found my own place to preserve her memory within my world. Of course one of her many pleasures in life were to eat and gather strawberries. At my own home I am with luck to have a wild strawberry patch just up the hill from my house. Whenever I am in need of her presence I just simply pace onward to the patch of land that she loved. There I can reminisce and be weepy or glad.

For all the families that have had to bond together in face of any tragedy, we can only do our best and hope that it may be enough. With patience and sacrifice, maybe we can make a difference.

Since Esther's passing the Haas daughters and their

families have made their way to Edmonton for the past four years to participate in the Spring Sprint for The Brain Tumor Foundation. We raise funds to help with research and education.

BECAUSE OF YOU MOM AND DAD

I AM ME

Because of you mom and dad

I know what being a family all is about.

We have learnt to live life and laugh along the way.

We have leaned on each other and bent when necessary.

We have found patience and we sacrifice for each other.

We are friends until the end, no matter what lies ahead.

Because of the two of you,

I know what is really at the heart of a good life.

It's simply family and the love that we feel.

I know all of this because of you

THE END

About the Author

Carmen Wurst (nee) Haas

My parents Ernie and Esther Haas raised their four daughters in Grimshaw. Alberta. My father along with my sisters and their families still reside there

I am blessed with a tall slender humorous, very pleasant and talented son. My other great gift in life is my beautiful caring nurturing and loyal daughter. My husband and I have been married for twenty six years.

I have lived in Bonnyville for the last fourteen years. We have run a Bed and Breakfast from our home on Moose Lake for the last nine years.

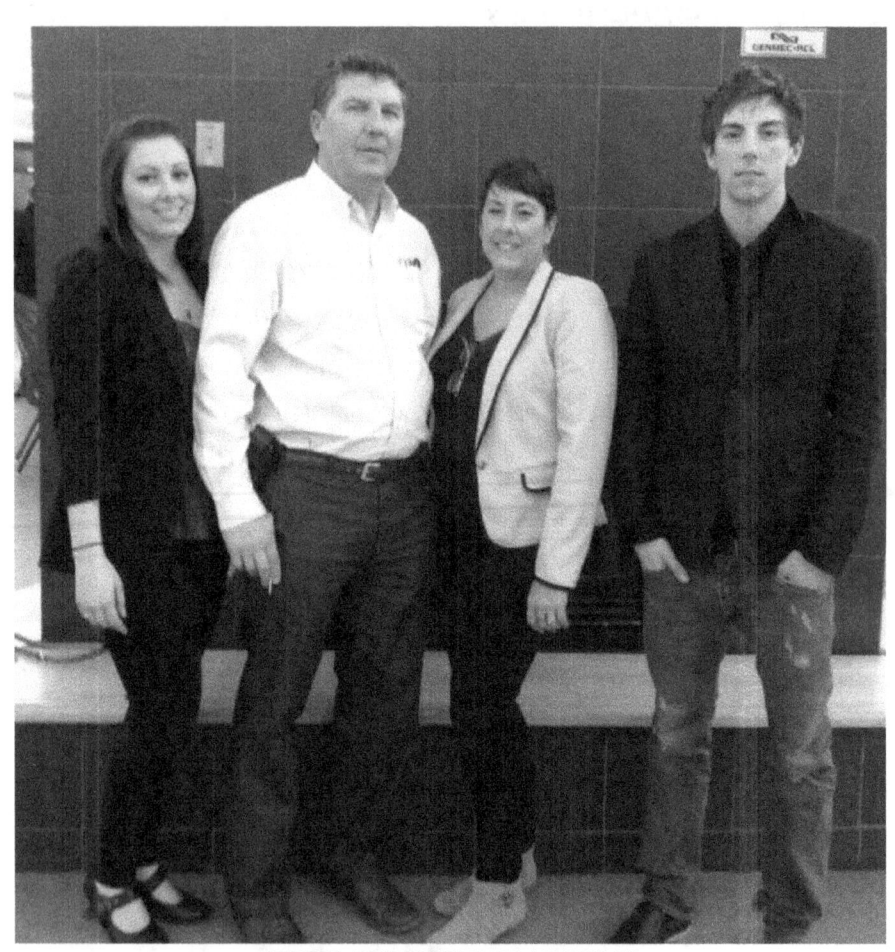

THE WURST FAMILY